Hip Dysplasia

Editors

TISHA A.M. HARPER
J. RYAN BUTLER

VETERINARY CLINICS OF NORTH AMERICA: SMALL ANIMAL PRACTICE

www.vetsmall.theclinics.com

July 2017 • Volume 47 • Number 4

ELSEVIER

1600 John F. Kennedy Boulevard • Suite 1800 • Philadelphia, Pennsylvania, 19103-2899
http://www.vetsmall.theclinics.com

**VETERINARY CLINICS OF NORTH AMERICA: SMALL ANIMAL PRACTICE Volume 47, Number 4
July 2017 ISSN 0195-5616, ISBN-13: 978-0-323-53160-3**

Editor: Katie Pfaff
Developmental Editor: Meredith Madeira

Photocopying

Single photocopies of single articles may be made for personal use as allowed by national copyright laws. Permission of the Publisher and payment of a fee is required for all other photocopying, including multiple or systematic copying, copying for advertising or promotional purposes, resale, and all forms of document delivery. Special rates are available for educational institutions that wish to make photocopies for non-profit educational classroom use. For information on how to seek permission visit www.elsevier.com/permissions or call: (+44) 1865 843830 (UK)/(+1) 215 239 3804 (USA).

Derivative Works

Subscribers may reproduce tables of contents or prepare lists of articles including abstracts for internal circulation within their institutions. Permission of the Publisher is required for resale or distribution outside the institution. Permission of the Publisher is required for all other derivative works, including compilations and translations (please consult www.elsevier.com/permissions).

Electronic Storage or Usage

Permission of the Publisher is required to store or use electronically any material contained in this periodical, including any article or part of an article (please consult www.elsevier.com/permissions). Except as outlined above, no part of this publication may be reproduced, stored in a retrieval system or transmitted in any form or by any means, electronic, mechanical, photocopying, recording or otherwise, without prior written permission of the Publisher.

Notice

No responsibility is assumed by the Publisher for any injury and/or damage to persons or property as a matter of products liability, negligence or otherwise, or from any use or operation of any methods, products, instructions or ideas contained in the material herein. Because of rapid advances in the medical sciences, in particular, independent verification of diagnoses and drug dosages should be made.

Although all advertising material is expected to conform to ethical (medical) standards, inclusion in this publication does not constitute a guarantee or endorsement of the quality or value of such product or of the claims made of it by its manufacturer.

Veterinary Clinics of North America: Small Animal Practice (ISSN 0195-5616) is published bimonthly by Elsevier Inc., 360 Park Avenue South, New York, NY 10010-1710. Months of issue are January, March, May, July, September, and November. Business and Editorial Offices: 1600 John F. Kennedy Blvd., Ste. 1800, Philadelphia, PA 19103-2899. Customer Service Office: 3251 Riverport Lane, Maryland Heights, MO 63043. Periodicals postage paid at New York, NY and additional mailing offices. Subscription prices are $319.00 per year (domestic individuals), $598.00 per year (domestic institutions), $100.00 per year (domestic students/residents), $422.00 per year (Canadian individuals), $743.00 per year (Canadian institutions), $469.00 per year (international individuals), $743.00 per year (international institutions), and $220.00 per year (international and Canadian students/residents). To receive student/resident rate, orders must be accompanied by name of affiliated institution, date of term, and the *signature* of program/residency coordinator on institution letterhead. Orders will be billed at individual rate until proof of status is received. Foreign air speed delivery is included in all *Clinics* subscription prices. All prices are subject to change without notice. **POSTMASTER:** Send address changes to *Veterinary Clinics of North America: Small Animal Practice*, Elsevier Health Sciences Division, Subscription Customer Service, 3251 Riverport Lane, Maryland Heights, MO 63043. Customer Service (orders, claims, online, change of address): Elsevier Periodicals Customer Service, Elsevier Health Sciences Division Subscription **Customer Service 3251 Riverport Lane Maryland Heights, MO 63043. Tel: 1-800-654-2452 (U.S. and Canada); 314-447-8871 (outside U.S. and Canada). Fax: 314-447-8029. E-mail: journalscustomerservice-usa@elsevier.com (for print support); journalsonlinesupport-usa@elsevier.com (for online support).**

Reprints. For copies of 100 or more of articles in this publication, please contact the Commercial Reprints Department, Elsevier Inc., 360 Park Avenue South, New York, NY 10010-1710. Tel.: 212-633-3874; Fax: 212-633-3820; E-mail: reprints@elsevier.com.

Veterinary Clinics of North America: Small Animal Practice is also published in Japanese by Inter Zoo Publishing Co., Ltd., Aoyama Crystal-Bldg 5F, 3-5-12 Kitaaoyama, Minato-ku, Tokyo 107-0061, Japan.

Veterinary Clinics of North America: Small Animal Practice is covered in *Current Contents/Agriculture, Biology and Environmental Sciences, Science Citation Index, ASCA, MEDLINE/PubMed (Index Medicus), Excerpta Medica, and BIOSIS.*

Contributors

EDITORS

TISHA A.M. HARPER, DVM, MS, CCRP
Diplomate, American College of Veterinary Surgeons–Small Animal; Clinical Assistant Professor, Small Animal Surgery, Department of Veterinary Clinical Medicine, University of Illinois College of Veterinary Medicine, Urbana, Illinois

J. RYAN BUTLER, DVM, MS
Diplomate, American College of Veterinary Surgeons–Small Animal; Assistant Professor, Small Animal Surgery, Department of Clinical Sciences, College of Veterinary Medicine, Mississippi State University, Mississippi State, Mississippi

AUTHORS

J. RYAN BUTLER, DVM, MS
Diplomate, American College of Veterinary Surgeons–Small Animal; Assistant Professor, Small Animal Surgery, Department of Clinical Sciences, College of Veterinary Medicine, Mississippi State University, Mississippi State, Mississippi

DAVID L. DYCUS, DVM, MS, CCRP
Diplomate, American College of Veterinary Surgeons–Small Animal; Department of Orthopedic Surgery, Veterinary Orthopedic and Sports Medicine Group (VOSM), Annapolis Junction, Maryland

SAMUEL P. FRANKLIN, MS, DVM, PhD
Diplomate, American College of Veterinary Surgeons–Small Animal; Diplomate, American College of Veterinary Sports Medicine and Rehabilitation; Assistant Professor, Small Animal Orthopedic Surgery, Department of Small Animal Medicine and Surgery, University of Georgia College of Veterinary Medicine, Athens, Georgia

JENNIFER GAMBINO, DVM
Diplomate, American College of Veterinary Radiology; Assistant Professor, Diagnostic Imaging, Department of Clinical Sciences, College of Veterinary Medicine, Mississippi State University, Mississippi State, Mississippi

FRANCISCO GUEVARA, DVM
Postdoctoral Orthopedic Research Fellow, Department of Small Animal Medicine and Surgery, University of Georgia College of Veterinary Medicine, Athens, Georgia

TISHA A.M. HARPER, DVM, MS, CCRP
Diplomate, American College of Veterinary Surgeons–Small Animal; Clinical Assistant Professor, Small Animal Surgery, Department of Veterinary Clinical Medicine, University of Illinois College of Veterinary Medicine, Urbana, Illinois

DAVID HUMMEL, DVM
Diplomate, American College of Veterinary Surgeons–Small Animal; Staff Surgeon, Department of Surgery, Skylos Sports Medicine, Ellicott City, Maryland and Frederick, Maryland

MICHAEL D. KING, BVSc, MS
Diplomate, American College of Veterinary Surgeons; Department of Surgery, Canada West Veterinary Specialists & Critical Care Hospital, Vancouver, British Columbia, Canada

DAVID LEVINE, PT, PhD, DPT, CCRP, Cert DN
Diplomate, American Board of Physical Therapy Specialists (Orthopedics); Department of Physical Therapy, University of Tennessee at Chattanooga, Chattanooga, Tennessee

KATHLEEN A. LINN, DVM, MS
Department of Small Animal Clinical Sciences, Western College of Veterinary Medicine, University of Saskatchewan, Saskatoon, Saskatchewan, Canada

DENIS J. MARCELLIN-LITTLE, DEDV
Diplomate, American College of Veterinary Surgeons; Diplomate, American College of Veterinary Sports Medicine and Rehabilitation; Department of Clinical Sciences, College of Veterinary Medicine, North Carolina State University, Raleigh, North Carolina

JENNIFER K. REAGAN, DVM
Diplomate, American College of Veterinary Surgeons–Small Animal; Department of Veterinary Clinical Medicine, University of Illinois College of Veterinary Medicine, Urbana, Illinois

TERESA D. SCHILLER, DVM
Diplomate, American College of Veterinary Surgeons; Associate Dean, Clinical Programs; Senior Instructor, Department of Veterinary Clinical and Diagnostic Services, University of Calgary, Faculty of Veterinary Medicine, Calgary, Alberta, Canada

JASON SYRCLE, DVM
Diplomate, American College of Veterinary Surgeons–Small Animal; Associate Clinical Professor, Small Animal Surgery, Department of Clinical Sciences, College of Veterinary Medicine, Mississippi State University, Mississippi State, Mississippi

Contents

Preface: Hip Dysplasia: Where Are We Now and How Do We Treat?   xi

Tisha A.M. Harper and J. Ryan Butler

Etiopathogenesis of Canine Hip Dysplasia, Prevalence, and Genetics   753

Michael D. King

> First identified in 1935, canine hip dysplasia is thought to be the most common orthopedic condition diagnosed in the dog. It is most prevalent in large and giant breed dogs, with a complex polygenic mode of inheritance, and relatively low heritability. External factors including caloric intake when growing have a significant effect on phenotypic expression. Initial joint laxity progresses to osteoarthritis due to subluxation and abnormal wearing. Selective breeding programs to attempt to decrease prevalence have shown modest results so far.

Hip Dysplasia: Clinical Signs and Physical Examination Findings   769

Jason Syrcle

> Hip dysplasia is a common developmental disorder of the dog, consisting of varying degrees of hip laxity, progressive remodeling of the structures of the hip, and subsequent development of osteoarthritis. It is a juvenile-onset condition, with clinical signs often first evident at 4 to 12 months of age. A tentative diagnosis of hip dysplasia can be made based on signalment, history, and physical examination findings. The Ortolani test is a valuable tool for identifying juvenile dogs affected with this condition. Further diagnostics can then be prioritized, contributing to prompt diagnosis and appropriate treatment.

Canine Hip Dysplasia: Diagnostic Imaging   777

J. Ryan Butler and Jennifer Gambino

> Diagnostic imaging is the principal method used to screen for and diagnose hip dysplasia in the canine patient. Multiple techniques are available, each having advantages, disadvantages, and limitations. Hip-extended radiography is the most used method and is best used as a screening tool and for assessment for osteoarthritis. Distraction radiographic methods such as the PennHip method allow for improved detection of laxity and improved ability to predict future osteoarthritis development. More advanced techniques such as MRI, although expensive and not widely available, may improve patient screening and allow for improved assessment of cartilage health.

Canine Hip Dysplasia Screening Within the United States: Pennsylvania Hip Improvement Program and Orthopedic Foundation for Animals Hip/Elbow Database   795

Jennifer K. Reagan

> Canine hip dysplasia (CHD) is a complex, polygenic disease radiographically associated with hip subluxation and development of osteoarthritis. Screening

programs have been established with the goal of hip improvement, with the most common in the United States being OFA hip scoring and the PennHIP method. When evaluating the single hip-extended view used by OFA versus the 3 radiographic views and associated distraction index (DI) used by Penn-HIP for CHD screening, the scientific evidence supports the use of the DI and PennHIP method. OFA scoring can be used to effect hip improvement, especially when incorporated into estimated breeding values.

Conservative Management of Hip Dysplasia   807

Tisha A.M. Harper

Hip dysplasia (HD) is a common orthopedic condition seen in small animal patients that leads to osteoarthritis of the coxofemoral joint. The disease can be managed conservatively or surgically. The goals of surgical treatment in the immature patient are to either prevent the clinical signs of HD or to prevent or slow the progression of osteoarthritis. In mature patients surgery is used as a salvage procedure to treat debilitating osteoarthritis. Conservative management can be used in dogs with mild or intermittent clinical signs and includes nutritional management and weight control, exercise modification, physical rehabilitation, pain management and disease-modifying agents.

Physical Rehabilitation for the Management of Canine Hip Dysplasia   823

David L. Dycus, David Levine, and Denis J. Marcellin-Little

Hip dysplasia is among the most common orthopedic conditions affecting dogs. Joint laxity is responsible for abnormal development of the femoral head and acetabulum, leading to excessive wear of the articular cartilage. Wear leads to secondary osteoarthritis. Rehabilitation is either conservative or after surgical management. Conservative rehabilitation therapies are directed at decreasing pain, improving hip range of motion (ROM), and building or maintaining muscle mass. Postoperatively, rehabilitation focuses on decreasing postoperative pain and inflammation, improving comfort and limb use, and protecting the surgical site. Once the patient has healed, rehabilitation is directed at improving ROM and promoting muscle mass.

Juvenile Pubic Symphysiodesis   851

Kathleen A. Linn

In properly selected dogs, juvenile pubic symphysiodesis improves joint congruity, decreases hip laxity, and can reverse or prevent progression of degenerative joint disease in the hips. To be effective, surgery must be done at a young age and in hips that are only mildly to moderately lax. Juvenile pubic symphysiodesis is best viewed more as a preemptive procedure than as a strictly therapeutic one. Dogs considered to be at risk for hip dysplasia should be screened with Ortolani testing at 12 weeks of age, with further imaging and perhaps surgery to follow for those who have a positive Ortolani sign.

Triple Pelvic Osteotomy and Double Pelvic Osteotomy   865

Francisco Guevara and Samuel P. Franklin

Triple and double pelvic osteotomy (TPO, DPO) are performed with the goal of increasing acetabular ventro-version, increasing femoral head coverage, and decreasing femoral head subluxation. Since the first descriptions of TPO, there have been modifications in technique, most notably omission of the ischial osteotomy for DPO, and improvements in the implants, including availability of locking TPO/DPO bone plates. Associated complication rates seem to have declined accordingly. The most salient questions regarding these procedures remain what selection criteria should be used to identify candidates and whether halting or preventing osteoarthritis is necessary to consider these surgeries clinically beneficial.

Femoral Head and Neck Excision 885

Tisha A.M. Harper

Femoral head and neck excision is a surgical procedure that is commonly performed in small animal patients. It is a salvage procedure that is done to relieve pain in the coxofemoral joint and restore acceptable function of the limb. Femoral head and neck excision is most commonly used to treat severe osteoarthritis in the coxofemoral joint and can be done in dogs and cats of any size or age. The procedure should not be overused and ideally should not be done when the integrity of the coxofemoral joint can be restored.

BioMedtrix Total Hip Replacement Systems: An Overview 899

Teresa D. Schiller

Total hip replacement for canine and feline patients affected by degenerative, traumatic, and vascular injury of the coxofemoral joint has become a highly successful orthopedic procedure. The highly effective BioMedtrix total hip replacement systems use cemented and cementless implants with unique design features to address a variety of bone conditions and surgeon expertise and preferences. There are pros and cons for both systems with common and unique complications that can occur in either system. Surgeon experience and adherence to the principles of technique will strongly influence the complication rate and outcomes.

Zurich Cementless Total Hip Replacement 917

David Hummel

Total hip replacement (THR) is the gold standard treatment of intractable pain from hip dysplasia. THR procedures are divided into 2 main categories: cemented and cementless, with hybrid a combination. The Zurich Cementless THR system uses a combination of press-fit (acetabular component) and locking screw (femoral component) fixation designed to address the main challenge facing cemented systems (aseptic loosening) while providing the benefit of immediate stability with its novel locking screw implantation system for the femoral stem. The Zurich THR system is an effective treatment option for orthopedic conditions of the coxofemoral joint in medium to giant breed dogs.

INNOPLANT Total Hip Replacement System 935

Tisha A.M. Harper

Total hip replacement is a salvage procedure that is done to alleviate discomfort secondary to osteoarthritis in the hip, which is most often a result of hip dysplasia. Commercially available total hip replacement implants for small animal patients are classified as cemented or cementless. The INNOPLANT Total Hip Replacement system includes modular, screw-in cementless components that were developed to improve implant stability by maintaining as much normal anatomic structure, and by extension biomechanics of the coxofemoral joint, as possible. As a newer system, there are few data and no long-term studies available in the veterinary literature.

Index   **945**

VETERINARY CLINICS OF NORTH AMERICA: SMALL ANIMAL PRACTICE

FORTHCOMING ISSUES

September 2017
Topics in Cardiology
Joao S. Orvalho, *Editor*

November 2017
Wound Management
Marije Risselada, *Editor*

January 2018
Neurology
Sharon C. Kerwin and Amanda R. Taylor, *Editors*

RECENT ISSUES

May 2017
Hepatology
Jonathan Lidbury, *Editor*

March 2017
Advances in Fluid, Electrolyte, and Acid-base Disorders
Helio Autran de Morais and Stephen P. DiBartola, *Editors*

January 2017
Cytology
Amy L. MacNeill, *Editor*

THE CLINICS ARE NOW AVAILABLE ONLINE!
Access your subscription at:
www.theclinics.com

Preface

Hip Dysplasia: Where Are We Now and How Do We Treat?

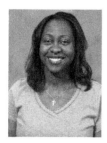 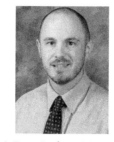

Tisha A.M. Harper, DVM, MS, CCRP   J. Ryan Butler, DVM, MS
Editors

Hip dysplasia is a common cause of hindlimb lameness in the dog and is a disease with which the veterinary practitioner is faced on a regular basis. The spectrum of clinical signs varies from asymptomatic to debilitating osteoarthritis and severe lameness. The goal of this issue is to present a comprehensive yet concise review of hip dysplasia from etiopathogenesis to treatment, highlighting the latest developments and treatment options available to the veterinary practitioner. The etiopathogenesis and hip dysplasia screening articles detail the work that has been done to determine the heritability of the disease and develop programs to decrease the incidence of the disease in the canine population. The disease is, however, still quite prevalent, and not much has changed with regard to clinical signs and presentation. The field of physical rehabilitation for dogs has grown by leaps and bounds in the last 15 to 20 years. In addition, there are many more pharmacologic options for managing the pain associated with osteoarthritis in the dysplastic pet. The conservative management and physical rehabilitation articles highlight pharmacologic options and many of the modalities, both passive and active, currently available for the nonsurgical management of hip dysplasia. They also highlight emerging treatment options such as stem cell therapy. The latter articles in this issue focus on many surgical options for the treatment of dogs with hip dysplasia. Some of these procedures have been around for many years but have been improved upon to diminish complications (eg, there have been many modifications to the original total hip replacement system, the BioMedtrix Total Hip Replacement System, to improve implant stability and decrease complications). There are other historical surgical procedures that have been described to treat hip dysplasia (eg, muscle sling procedures, intertrochanteric femoral osteotomy) that have fallen out of favor in lieu of newer techniques with more predictable outcomes. However, we would be remiss if we did not acknowledge the contributions of these pioneers.

Vet Clin Small Anim 47 (2017) xi–xii
http://dx.doi.org/10.1016/j.cvsm.2017.04.001
0195-5616/17/© 2017 Published by Elsevier Inc.   **vetsmall.theclinics.com**

This is our first foray as editors, and we are grateful for this opportunity. We would like to thank the group of authors who have contributed to this issue, and we hope that it will sit prominently on your library shelves and serve as a ready reference.

Tisha A.M. Harper, DVM, MS, CCRP
Department of Veterinary Clinical Medicine
College of Veterinary Medicine
University of Illinois at Urbana-Champaign
1008 West Hazelwood Drive
MC 004
Urbana, IL 61802, USA

J. Ryan Butler, DVM, MS
Department of Clinical Sciences
College of Veterinary Medicine
Mississippi State University
240 Wise Center Drive
Mississippi State, MS 39762, USA

E-mail addresses:
taharper@illinois.edu (T.A.M. Harper)
ryan.butler@msstate.edu (J.R. Butler)

Etiopathogenesis of Canine Hip Dysplasia, Prevalence, and Genetics

Michael D. King, BVSc, MS

KEYWORDS

- Pathogenesis • Genetic • Dysplasia • Prevalence

KEY POINTS

- Canine hip dysplasia is the most common orthopedic condition diagnosed in the dog, with prevalence of up to 71% in affected breeds.
- As a polygenic genetic disease, it has a complex mode of inheritance, with phenotypic expression affected by external factors.
- Joint laxity leads to abnormal wearing of the coxofemoral joint and subsequent osteoarthritis.
- Although some specific genes that contribute to hip dysplasia have been identified, the basis for hip dysplasia consists of many genes each contributing a small effect.

INTRODUCTION

First described in 1935 by Schnelle, canine hip dysplasia (CHD) is considered to be the most common orthopedic condition diagnosed in the dog.[1–7] As most patients have only mild clinical signs associated with CHD, it is possible, however, that cranial cruciate ligament rupture is a more common cause of hind limb lameness.[8,9] Even in dogs with only minor radiographic evidence of CHD, a change in gait is often present despite the lack of an obvious lameness.[10]

CHD has a genetic basis, although with a polygenic or complex mode of inheritance. Multiple environmental factors modify the expression of this predisposition, affecting the way it manifests, and its severity.[1,2,4,5,11–15] Although seen in a variety of breeds, CHD is most prevalent in large, fast-growing dogs, with Labrador retrievers, Newfoundlands, rottweilers, St. Bernards, and mastiffs commonly affected. Bulldogs, pugs, and some terrier breeds are also very predisposed.[3–5,16]

Disclosure: The author has nothing to disclose.
Department of Surgery, Canada West Veterinary Specialists & Critical Care Hospital, 1988 Kootenay Street, Vancouver, British Columbia V5M 4Y3, Canada
E-mail address: mking@canadawestvets.com

Vet Clin Small Anim 47 (2017) 753–767
http://dx.doi.org/10.1016/j.cvsm.2017.03.001
vetsmall.theclinics.com

CAUSE

The exact cause of CHD remains unknown, although it was defined by Henricson in 1966 as "a varying degree of laxity of the hip joint permitting subluxation during early life, giving rise to varying degrees of shallow acetabulum and flattening of the femoral head, finally, inevitably leading to osteoarthritis."[14] The phenotypic expression of a genetically predisposed dog is joint laxity, which is the focus of both early diagnostics and traditional screening techniques, as well as some surgical treatment methods in young patients.[1–4,17,18] However, joint laxity alone, although necessary, does not seem to be sufficient in isolation for the development of CHD.[19,20] There appears to be significant breed and individual variation in the tolerance of a specific degree of joint laxity, and both the rate and the incidence of subsequent development of osteoarthritis (OA).[20–22]

Although CHD is considered (by definition) to be a disease of the coxofemoral joints, there is evidence that this may be the most visible aspect of a more generalized disease in predisposed dogs. It is known that puppies that develop with excessive joint laxity in the hips have a high risk of developing OA in those joints later in life.[1,3,17,19,23,24] However, they are also at increased risk of developing OA of the shoulder, and potentially other joints, including the elbow, stifle, vertebra, and mandibular joint.[4,25] One study identified increased cartilage weights, and increased fibronectin content of cartilage sampled from the humerus in dogs with CHD, which are thought to be early indicators of OA.[26]

PATHOGENESIS

Dogs predisposed to CHD are born with normal hips that subsequently become dysplastic, exhibiting increased joint laxity. The reason for this remains unclear, although abnormalities in endochondral ossification and acetabular development are also thought to be involved.[1,27]

Joint Laxity

Passive hip joint laxity is that which is able to be measured by palpation or sedated radiograph and may be tolerated by individuals without any apparent dysfunction. Functional laxity is the pathologic instability that actually occurs during weight-bearing, resulting in subluxation of the femoral head and abnormal forces across the joint. It cannot be measured directly, and passive laxity is used as an approximation.[1,3,28]

Primary anatomic stabilizers of the coxofemoral joint include the ligament of the head of the femur, the joint capsule, and the dorsal acetabular rim.[29] The synovial fluid, in combination with the joint capsule, also provides a powerful stabilizing effect.[5,23]

The ligament of the head of the femur has been shown to be abnormal and thickened in dogs with dysplastic hips exhibiting moderate to severe OA.[30] A later study however showed no such difference in the volume of the ligament in dogs with mild OA.[31]

Joint stability in neutral positions is maintained in large part due to atmospheric pressures, through the vacuum phenomenon within the joint itself.[3,23] A close association has been demonstrated between the volume of synovial fluid present and the degree of laxity within the hip, with increased fluid resulting in more pronounced laxity, and vice versa.[4,32] Increased joint fluid volumes have been confirmed within the coxofemoral joints of dogs exhibiting CHD, which has led to some suggestion that hip laxity could be secondary to excessive synovial fluid quantities. The fact that this volume (as measured by the distraction index [DI]) remains constant through early periods of development is surmised by some investigators as evidence of this.[1,4,23]

Synovial fluid is mainly created through dialysis of blood within the intracapsular vessels, with plasma modified by vascular endothelium, connective tissue, and synoviocytes. There are no known active homeostatic mechanisms in synovial fluid regulation, with removal through intracapsular veins and lymphatics maintaining a balance.[23] Inflammatory processes can affect this balance, with leakage of proteins into the joint and decreasing drainage. In addition, as intraarticular pressure increases, synoviocytes decrease in size, which enlarges intercellular gaps, contributing to greater permeability of the joint capsule, further increasing joint fluid accumulation.[23,31] These factors make it uncertain if increased joint fluid within the coxofemoral joint of a dog with CHD is a primary cause of joint laxity, or if it is simply synovitis as a result of that laxity.

The mechanical strength of the joint capsule is determined by its collagen content, something that is known to be abnormal in people with hip dysplasia. One study investigated the ratio of type III:I collagen in coxofemoral joint synovium, with a high ratio indicating a weak joint capsule, because type I collagen is needed for strength. This study showed an increased ratio in breeds predisposed to CHD compared with greyhounds, although no difference between dysplastic and nondysplastic dogs in each group.[33] A follow-up study assessed the same ratio in the umbilical tissues of newborn puppies, which showed no difference between dysplastic and nondysplastic dogs.[23] The investigators concluded that this did not support a primary, generalized alteration in collagen composition in dysplastic dogs.

Subluxation

Traditionally it has been thought that subluxation occurs with weight-bearing (functional laxity), and the femoral head in a dysplastic hip then translates laterally. The muscle forces acting around the hip increase, whereas the contact area within the hip decreases, resulting in incongruence and abnormal wearing of articular cartilage.[1,3,19]

An alternative theory has been proposed to explain the pathogenic mechanism of joint laxity causing joint degeneration in dogs with CHD; the investigators surmise that subluxation is occurring during the swing phase of the gait, rather than upon weight-bearing. With normal (low) levels of synovial fluid, any lateral translation of the femoral head during the swing phase of ambulation would result in invagination and stretching of the joint capsule. Mechanoreceptors within the capsule would then be triggered, recruiting adjacent muscles to contract in a protective role, positioning the femoral head closer to the acetabulum. With increased synovial fluid present, it would theoretically take more pronounced subluxation of the femoral head during the swing phase to trigger the same stretch response and muscle recruitment. Upon weight-bearing, the hip would be positioned in a progressively more subluxated orientation, leading to sudden and damaging reduction of the hip.[1]

Although not proven, their justification of this lies in the distribution and action of muscles around the hip. During weight-bearing, several powerful muscles (specifically the gluteals and adductors), oriented largely perpendicular to the joint, act together providing a strong resolved force directing the femoral head into a reduced position within the acetabulum. In contrast, during the swing phase, the muscles involved in advancing the limb (iliopsoas, rectus femoris, sartorius) produce a weaker force, but oriented parallel to the femur, creating a net vertical load that predisposes to hip subluxation. In addition, the investigators propose that if subluxation and abnormal wearing occurred during weight-bearing, cartilage damage would be focused more cranially in the femoral head and acetabulum, in line with the strongest propulsive forces. They note that the characteristic location and distribution of cartilage wear are immediately dorsal to the fovea capitis, suggesting it is "catastrophic reduction" of the femoral head upon weight-bearing causing joint degeneration.[1]

Alterations in endochondral ossification in the developing pelvis have also been proposed as a contributor to CHD.[2] The acetabulum forms between the ventral arms of the shared physis of the ilium, pubis, and ischium, known as the triradiate growth plate. A secondary acetabular ossification center then forms within the physis itself before closure at 4 to 5 months of age, whereas the capital physis closes between 9 and 11 months of age. Closure of the femoral capital physis has been shown to be delayed in dysplastic dogs, as is the onset of ossification of the femoral head.[2,34] This is thought to be due to compressive weight-bearing forces applied to the medial aspect of the femoral head and dorsal rim of the acetabulum interfering with normal ossification.[4]

Biomechanical factors associated with bone conformation in the pelvis have been proposed as contributing factors to CHD. Although femoral angle and degree of anteversion do not appear to have an effect, a steeper or more pronounced acetabular slope has been associated with subluxation.[19] This makes sense given the dorsal acetabular rim's role as a primary hip stabilizer, although it is uncertain if an increased acetabular slope is a primary factor, or if it occurs secondary to interference with normal hip development caused by joint laxity and abnormal wearing.

Lumbosacral abnormalities have also been shown to be somewhat associated with development of CHD, presumably due to the proximity to the developing pelvis.[35]

Normal force, congruency, and load are needed between the femoral head and acetabulum in order for the coxofemoral joint to develop correctly.

With hip subluxation, there is a concentration of mechanical load on the dorsal acetabular rim that may act to slow cartilage growth and development. The period of maximal growth and hip development occurs between 3 and 8 months of age in dogs, and abnormal forces at this age in a dysplastic hip are thought to have a critical effect on the expression of CHD in predisposed dogs.[2,3,19,36] Radiographic evidence of hip laxity can be seen as early as 2 months of age (although this has not always been shown to be strongly associated with development of CHD), with signs of OA identified sometime after 4 to 6 months of age.[3,14,22,28,32] Assessment of hip subluxation on a hip-extended ventrodorsal view radiograph has been the traditional method of diagnosis of CHD, with it the thought that dogs with apparently normal conformation by 2 years of age did not go on to develop significant degenerative joint disease. This has since been shown to be somewhat inaccurate, at least in part due to the technique's positioning artificially improving joint tightness. The DI radiographic technique has demonstrated accurate prediction of susceptibility to OA due to CHD, confirming joint laxity as the precursor to degenerative joint disease.[3,5,17,37]

Development of Osteoarthritis

Although hip laxity and subluxation in young dogs with CHD are seen to cause lameness in some individuals, it is the development of OA secondary to this laxity (or potentially with contribution from a separate genetic effect distinct from expression of CHD) that causes the most morbidity.[3–5,21] Development of OA has traditionally been described as a biphasic, seen most often before 2 years of age, and then again when geriatric, but is now thought to progress with a more linear incidence as dogs age.[3]

Clinical signs are seen in juvenile dogs with tearing and inflammation of the joint capsule, as well as microfracture of the dorsal acetabular rim.[1,4,38] In response to this damage, periarticular fibrosis forms and is associated with a decreased incidence of clinical signs. It was initially thought that the fibrosis results in increased joint stability, although this is questionable, with a more recent study demonstrating increasing laxity with progression of OA.[39]

Whatever the exact mechanism, hip laxity and subluxation result in incongruence of the coxofemoral joint, and increased force acting over a smaller contact area. This causes abnormal wearing of the cartilage, and microfractures of the dorsal acetabular rim.[1,4,38] The degree of laxity and remodeling present at 6 months, as assessed by the reduction angle of the hip, have been shown to be a strong predictor of OA development at 2 years of age.[19]

Initial stress on articular cartilage results in release of destructive enzymes from chondrocytes, synoviocytes, and inflammatory cells that degrade matrix proteoglycans.[40] Water content within the cartilage increases, and damage to underlying collagen structure occurs, leading to fibrillation and decreased cartilage stiffness, making it more susceptible to injury.[31,38,40] Because of this biomechanical change, the cartilage is subjected to increased strain (greater deformation when a load is applied) and is less able to return to its normal shape once the load is released.[38] Inflammatory cytokines, such as inerleukin-1 (IL-1), IL-6, and tumor necrosis factor, are known to be involved in this process and have been confirmed to be present in increased amounts in the hips of dysplastic dogs.[31,41]

Microfractures and stress on the subchondral bone occur due to abnormal weight-bearing on the femoral head and dorsal acetabular rim. As it remodels and heals, the bone at both sites becomes denser and less able to absorb shock. A larger amount of the weight-bearing force is then transmitted to the overlying cartilage, accelerating degeneration.[2,4,42]

Synovial fluid loses some viscosity due to lower hyaluronan content, which decreases joint lubrication. Fragments of damaged cartilage worsen the inflammatory response, creating further chondrocyte loss.[40]

Proliferation of chondrocytes occurs, in an attempt to compensate for damage. They form clusters of cells, often at the edge of the lesion.[2] This cartilage synthesis is associated with greater cartilage thickness, due to tissue swelling as well as an increase in both number of cells and amount of extracellular matrix. Although there is initially an upregulation of degradation and synthesis processes, eventually the cartilage is unable to maintain its repair processes, and chondrocyte loss occurs.[4,23,31]

Subchondral bone becomes exposed, resulting in yet further inflammation. Through weight-bearing and remodeling, it becomes sclerotic and eburnated with a polished appearance.[4,38,40] Focal subchondral bone necrosis occurs, thought to be due to heat caused by friction or repeated microfracture.[38]

Continued inflammation and abnormal wearing create additional loss of normal joint conformation. The acetabulum becomes shallower and wider, whereas the femoral head flattens.[1,4,38] Increased stress and inflammation of the synovium result in tearing of Sharpey fibers at the insertion of the joint capsule, which sees the formation of osteophytes.[4,38,40] Mesenchymal stem cells within the periosteum or synovial lining are thought to be the precursors of true osteophytes at the joint margin,[40] with cytokines of the transforming growth factor-beta family (TGF-ß) also involved in the induction of osteophytosis. Injection of TGF-ß into experimentally normal joints has resulted in osteophyte formation, and its expression has been identified in osteophytes from both people and animals with OA.[31] As osteophytosis and bone remodeling progress, the characteristic radiographic appearance of thickening of the femoral neck and proliferation of the dorsal acetabular rim is seen.[4,5,38]

OA is an irreversible outcome of CHD and can be extremely debilitating. Although most dogs with CHD exhibit no or only mild clinical signs, its high prevalence makes it a very serious problem, especially as many of the breeds commonly affected are highly trained working and service dogs.[4,43] Because there is no definitive therapy for OA, improving patient welfare requires better understanding of the genetic basis of CHD, it is hoped, to decrease the prevalence in affected breeds through selective breeding.[4,12,43]

GENETICS

Two factors determine the expression of CHD in a dog: genetic predisposition and environment. An individual's phenotype (whether they exhibit hip laxity and CHD) is determined by its genotype in combination with influencing external environmental factors.[2,4,12]

Heritability

The degree to which the expression of a condition is explained by its genotype is quantified by the estimate of the trait's heritability, which is designated by the symbol h^2. Heritability is defined as the ratio of additive genetic variation:the overall phenotypic variation of a given trait ($h^2 = V_g/V_p$).[4,12] Therefore, a heritability of 1.0 indicates that the occurrence of the trait is entirely controlled by the presence or absence of a gene, regardless of any environmental factors. A heritability of 0.0 means the trait is not genetically influenced. CHD is a polygenic trait, influenced by environmental effects.[4,12] Polygenic inheritance implies a large, but unknown number of alleles involved, scattered throughout the genome.[44,45]

The heritability of CHD has been estimated between 0.1 and 0.6, with most values decreasing to less than 0.5.[2,4,11,12,43,44,46] A large study assessing hip scores for Labrador retrievers in the United Kingdom identified heritability of 0.34 from the parents, with 0.41 from the sire alone and 0.3 from the dam alone.[46] A study of more than 1700 boxers from 325 litters identified a heritability of only 0.11 for development of clinical signs of CHD.[43] Two early studies assessing German shepherds identified heritability estimates of 0.22 and 0.43 for subjective hip scores.[12] A more recent investigation of 4 less common breeds found the pooled heritability for hip scores in English setters, Portuguese water dogs, Chinese shar peis, and Bernese mountain dogs as 0.26.[47]

These estimates would be considered to show low heritability, because any genetic change would be slow with selective breeding.[12]

As heritability is specific to the population of dogs being investigated, it is also specific to the trait being assessed.[11,12] Coxofemoral joint laxity has been shown to demonstrate higher levels of heritability than hip scoring. Heritability estimates for laxity of 0.46 in German shepherds and Labrador retrievers, 0.64 in golden retrievers, and 0.85 in Estrela mountain dogs have been described.[11,12] A study that assessed dogs from 17 different breeds identified heritability estimates of 0.61 for the DI and 0.73 for the Norberg angle.[48] This is important, because the higher the heritability of a trait, the greater the expected genetic improvement over time from selective breeding.

Selection Pressure

Breeding parents with a phenotype that is better than the average for the population overall exerts a selection pressure on the progeny. The selection pressure is determined as the difference between the average phenotype of the parents and the average phenotype of the population. The expected genetic change, or improvement in average phenotype of the progeny (ΔG), can be calculated as follows:

$\Delta G = h^2 \times (\text{Average}_{\text{parents}} - \text{Average}_{\text{population}})$

The amount of genetic change expected is therefore dependent on the heritability of the trait, and the amount of selection pressure able to be applied.[12] As an example, if one considers the DI in a breeding pair and assumes a heritability of 0.25, with a parental average of 0.2, and a population average of 0.6, the following formula results:

$\Delta G = 0.25 \times -0.4$

$\Delta G = -0.1$

Thus, the low heritability in this example leads to only 25% of the selection pressure being applied and results in a slow rate of genetic improvement. In addition, as the difference between the population average and the average of the selected parents becomes less pronounced with each generation, the amount of selection pressure able to be applied decreases. Therefore, progress over time becomes more incremental as prevalence decreases.[4,11,12]

Traditional selective breeding schemes have used hip scores based on the ventrodorsal extended-hip-view radiograph, with in general only slow genetic improvement shown over time.[1] A study of German shepherds in Finland showed no genetic improvement when using subjective hip scores as criteria.[49] Assessment of the progress of 6 breeds within the UK screening system showed no significant improvement in genetic progress over 13 years, and in the case of the Siberian husky, the hip scores had in fact worsened slightly.[50] A more recent investigation of UK dogs also identified a worsening genetic trend for CHD in the Siberian husky.[43] Because the husky has traditionally had extremely good hip scores, it is hypothesized that as a sled dog the breed had undergone selection against lameness (including CHD), but with increasing popularity as a pet and as show dogs, that this selection pressure may have weakened.

A US study of dogs assessed through the Orthopedic Foundation for Animals (OFA) scoring system identified significant improvement in hip scores.[51] An investigation of specifically Labrador retrievers within the OFA system also identified improvement over time, although it was minimal. This study identified a low heritability of only 0.21, which may explain the slow progress.[52]

Applying selection pressure based on other traits with higher heritability, such as DI, or dorsolateral subluxation would be expected to improve the rate of genetic improvement.[1,11,37]

Alternatively, the use of estimated breeding values (EBV) has been recommended to achieve even faster genetic progress.[1,11,12,44,48,53] An EBV is an assessment based on an individual's pedigree, derived from the hip quality of relatives and offspring. It is a more precise determination of a dog's genetic quality than individual records alone.[11] The EBV is calculated on a trait-by-trait basis for each dog and calculated to obtain a best linear unbiased prediction of a dog's relative genotype.[44,48] This calculation is then used to compare dogs for more accurate selection as potential breeding. Although time intensive, it has been shown to result in more rapid genetic improvement, with one study showing a decreased incidence of CHD in German shepherds from 55% to 24%, and in Labrador retrievers from 30% to 10%, in less than 5 generations.[44]

Genotyping

As with any inherited disease, the ideal technique for selective breeding and diagnosis would be a genetic test for the mutations that cause CHD. Inheritance of specific traits associated with CHD has been described, including femoral capital physeal ossification, DI, and subluxation score.[54] Unfortunately, because of the complex nature of the underlying genetics, progress in identifying specific genes or markers has been slow.[1,55,56]

A region on a chromosome that contains a gene or group of genes that influences the phenotypic expression of a quantitative trait such as CHD is referred to as a quantitative trait locus (QTL).[1,55] Several QTLs have been identified on several chromosomes, including on canine familiaris autosomes (CFAs) 01, 03, 04, 08, 09, 16, 19, 26, and 33,[57] and CFAs 04, 09, 10, 11, 16, 20, 22, 25, 29, 30, 35, and 37.[58] The identification of QTL in several studies in a variety of breeds suggests that at least 1 QTL on each of several chromosomes (CFAs 01, 04, 09, and 16) affects hip joint conformation.[59]

A specific QTL associated with acetabular osteophyte formation secondary to CHD in Portuguese water dogs has been identified on CFA 03.[60] This is thought to be evidence of QTLs that regulate the severity of secondary hip OA separately from those involved in expression of CHD.[21]

Recently, a fibrillar 2 gene haplotype (FBN2) was identified on CFA 11 associated with CHD. Dogs with the deletion haplotype exhibited significantly worse CHD as measured via DI, Norberg angle, extended hip radiograph, and dorsal subluxation score. FBN2 encodes for a component of extracellular matrix that is present in joint capsule and articular cartilage. Mutations of this gene have been associated with joint laxity in people.[61]

Only a small portion of the complex genetic basis for CHD has been determined so far and appears to consist of many genes that each contribute a small or moderate effect. This suggests that genomic selection, rather than specific marker-assisted selection, may be the most effective strategy for decreasing CHD prevalence.[62] There remains optimism that genotyping will eventually allow early intervention and improved selective breeding, and research is ongoing with the goal of developing accurate genetic screening for CHD.[56,63,64]

ENVIRONMENTAL FACTORS

Although an individual may be born with a genotypic predisposition to CHD, that does not automatically result in development of the condition. External factors do not cause hip dysplasia, but they determine whether CHD is expressed, and to what degree (**Table 1**).[4]

Nutrition

Two studies following a cohort of Labrador retrievers in the 1990s showed that limiting food consumption to 75% of that fed to control dogs from 8 weeks of age resulted in a 67% reduction in the prevalence of hip dysplasia at 2 years of age and substantially

Table 1	
External factors affecting expression of canine hip dysplasia	
Environmental Effects	
Risk factors	Protective Factors
Excessive food consumption	Limited food consumption
Rapid weight gain	Early off-leash exercise
Calcium supplementation	Glycosaminoglycan polysulfates
Dietary anion gap	
Early neuter	

reduced the prevalence and severity of hip joint OA at 5 years of age.[65,66] A follow-up study in 2000 confirmed the prevalence and severity of OA in several joints was less in dogs with long-term reduced food intake, compared with controls.[67]

Rapid weight gain has been determined to be a risk factor in some studies, especially when occurring within the first 6 months.[4,14,65] However, others have found no effect on joint laxity, or expression of CHD.[68,69] One investigation of 4 large breeds in Norway actually identified a protective effect of greater body weight at 3 months of age.[68]

Vitamin C is important in the development of collagen, and supplementing puppies and their dams with high doses was suspected to prevent CHD. There is no evidence that this is effective, and excessive vitamin C can interfere with normal bone and cartilage development. Dogs do not require dietary vitamin C, because they synthesize it themselves, so supplementation is not recommended.[4]

Puppies do not have a mechanism to protect against excess dietary calcium. Supplementing additional calcium or vitamin D results in decreased osteoclastic activity, delaying normal ossification, and can cause CHD in predisposed puppies.[1,2,4,70]

One study assessed the electrolyte balance of the diets fed to 167 dogs during a period of rapid growth. The investigators determined that on average significantly less subluxation of the femoral head was observed when diets with lower dietary anion gap were fed, and this was unrelated to growth rate.[71] This effect on subluxation is thought to be related to a decrease in synovial fluid volume associated with the low anion-gap diets.

Exercise

A correlation between pelvic muscle size and CHD has been described, with less muscle mass seen in dysplastic dogs compared with nondysplastic dogs.[72] Pelvic muscle mass indices (total postmortem mass of pelvic muscle [kg]/body weight [kg] $\times$ 100%) correctly predicted the presence of CHD 94% of the time. The disease was not present if the index was greater than 12 and consistently present when less than 9. Atrophy associated with CHD and early muscle conditioning did not seem to affect the index.

An investigation of risk factors for development of CHD in 4 large breeds in Norway identified that puppies walking on stairs from birth to 3 months of age had an increased incidence. However, they also identified off-leash activity through the same time period as having a protective effect. In addition, birth on a farm and birth in spring and summer resulted in a decreased risk of developing CHD. The investigators proposed that off-leash exercise (and being born into an environment and season that permits that) early in life may result in increased muscle development and strength in the hip area.[13]

The role of exercise in expression of CHD has not been as thoroughly investigated as nutrition, and further research is needed.[4]

Hormones

Several hormones have been proposed as potential contributors to CHD development. Estrogen, relaxin, insulin, and parathyroid hormone have all been investigated.[4] Estrogen administered to puppies has been shown to cause CHD. However, endogenous estrogen levels in dysplastic puppies are no higher than in nondysplastic animals.[1,2,4] Similarly, relaxin given to puppies can promote development of CHD.[1,2,4] Although there is no definitive evidence that endogenous relaxin causes CHD, higher and more persistent levels were identified in a group of lactating Labrador retrievers when compared with beagles. This finding may suggest an involvement in the higher prevalence of CHD seen in Labrador retrievers.[73]

An investigation of early-age neutering of male and female dogs identified a significant increase in the risk of developing CHD.[15] Assessment of more than 1800 dogs showed that of dogs neutered before 5.5 months of age, 6.7% developed CHD, whereas 4.7% of those neutered at or after 5.5 months of age developed CHD. However, those that were neutered at or after 5.5 months and developed CHD were 3 times more likely to be euthanized for the condition, compared with dogs that were neutered before 5.5 months of age and developed CHD.

Glycosaminoglycan Polysulfates

The only other treatment shown to have an effect on expression of CHD is administration of glycosaminoglycan polysulfates.[74] Twice weekly injections of 5 mg/kg were administered to CHD-susceptible puppies from 6 weeks to 8 months of age. Of the 8 puppies in the treated group, none showed signs of femoral head subluxation at 8 months, whereas 4 of 8 puppies in the control group did.

PREVALENCE

The overall prevalence of CHD in the canine population is unknown. An estimate made at a veterinary teaching hospital based on patients radiographed over a 5-year period determined prevalence within pure-breed dogs as 19.7%, and mix-breed dogs at 17.7%.[75] A more recent study assessed medical records from 27 veterinary teaching hospitals and showed a much lower prevalence of only 3.5%.[76] The investigators noted an increase in prevalence over time in their study but suspect this was due to increased recognition and diagnosis by veterinarians, rather than a true finding.

Prevalence of CHD between different breeds is extremely variable, ranging from 1% for some sighthounds to 71% for bulldogs[16] (**Fig. 1**). Reported prevalence within breeds is also often wide ranging, with numbers for golden retrievers ranging from 9.3% to 73%, and in rottweilers ranging from 11.8% to 53%.[16,76,77] The disparity is attributable to the difficulty in accurately assessing a truly representative sample of the total population, along with differences in prevalence between localized groups resulting in sampling bias.[2,77]

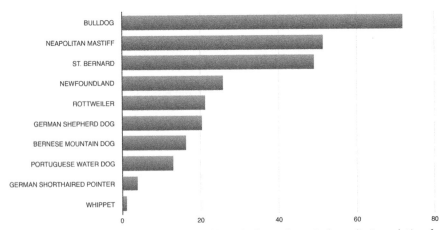

Fig. 1. Prevalence of CHD in a selection of breeds. (*Data from* Orthopedic Foundation for Animals. Available at: http://www.ofa.org/stats_hip.html.)

The only frequently updated and readily available data on CHD prevalence for multiple breeds in the United States is provided by the OFA through their radiographic screening program.[77] Although valuable, these data may underestimate true prevalence. As the OFA does not have a mandatory radiograph submission policy, prescreening by veterinarians is suspected to result in several films with obvious CHD never being assessed.[2,77] In addition, the OFA ventrodorsal radiograph view has been shown to underestimate CHD, and susceptibility to development of OA, when compared with other determinations of joint laxity such as DI.[78]

It is known that in general large and giant breeds have a higher prevalence of CHD, and castrated male dogs have also been identified to be more likely to exhibit the condition.[76] Specific breeds that are known to have a higher risk of CHD include Bernese mountain dog, Chesapeake Bay retriever, German shepherd, golden retriever, Labrador retriever, Newfoundland, old English sheep dog, rottweiler, St. Bernard, and Samoyed.[76,79] Conversely, some breeds identified as being at a lower risk include miniature schnauzer, Chihuahua, Maltese, toy poodle, dachshund.[76]

Despite the challenges in obtaining an accurate assessment of CHD prevalence in the canine population, it is clear that prevalence is unacceptably high in many breeds. Given the lack of effective treatments for resolving CHD once it occurs, continued efforts toward decreasing the prevalence through targeted breeding are needed.[77]

REFERENCES

1. Smith GK, Karbe GT, Agnello KA, et al. Pathogenesis, diagnosis, and control of canine hip dysplasia. In: Tobias KM, Johnston SA, editors. Veterinary surgery small animal, vol. 1, 1st edition. St Louis (MO): Elsevier; 2012. p. 824–48.

2. Krotscheck U, Tohundter T. Pathogenesis of hip dysplasia. In: Bojrab MJ, Monnet E, editors. Mechanisms of disease in small animal surgery. 3rd edition. Jackson (WY): Teton NewMedia; 2010. p. 636–45.

3. Kapatkin A, Fordyce H, Mayhew P, et al. Canine hip dysplasia: the disease and its diagnosis. Comp Cont Edu Pract Vet 2002;24:526–38.

4. Fries CL, Remedios AM. The pathogenesis and diagnosis of canine hip dysplasia: a review. Can Vet J 1995;36(8):494–502.

5. Brass W. Hip dysplasia in dogs. J Small Anim Pract 1989;30:166–70.

6. Lust G. An overview of the pathogenesis of canine hip dysplasia. J Am Vet Med Assoc 1997;210:1443–5.

7. Johnson J, Austin C, Breur G. Incidence of canine appendicular musculoskeletal disorders in 16 veterinary teaching hospitals from 1980 through 1989. Vet Comp Orthop Traumatol 1994;7:56–69.

8. Powers MY, Martinez SA, Lincoln JD, et al. Prevalence of cranial cruciate ligament rupture in a population of dogs with lameness previously attributed to hip dysplasia: 369 cases (1994-2003). J Am Vet Med Assoc 2005;227:1109–11.

9. Banfield CM, Bartels JE, Hudson JA, et al. A retrospective study of canine hip dysplasia in 116 military working dogs. Part II: clinical signs and performance data. J Am Anim Hosp Assoc 1996;32:423–30.

10. Bockstahler BA, Henninger W, Müller M, et al. Influence of borderline hip dysplasia on joint kinematics of clinically sound Belgian shepherd dogs. Am J Vet Res 2007;68:271–6.

11. Ginja MMD, Silvestre AM, Gonzalo-Orden JM, et al. Diagnosis, genetic control and preventive management of canine hip dysplasia: a review. Vet J 2010;184:269–76.

12. Kapatkin A, Mayhew P, Smith G. Genetic control of canine hip dysplasia. Comp Cont Edu Pract Vet 2002;24:681–7.

13. Krontveit RI, Nødtvedt A, Sævik BK, et al. Housing- and exercise-related risk factors associated with the development of hip dysplasia as determined by radiographic evaluation in a prospective cohort of Newfoundlands, Labrador retrievers, Leonbergers, and Irish wolfhounds in Norway. Am J Vet Res 2012; 73:838–46.

14. Richardson DC. The role of nutrition in canine hip dysplasia. Vet Clin North Am Small Anim Pract 1992;22:529–40.

15. Spain C, Scarlett J, Houpt K. Long-term risks and benefits of early-age gonadectomy in dogs. J Am Vet Med Assoc 2004;224:380–7.

16. Hip dysplasia by breed (Orthopedic Foundation Association data). Available at: http://ofa.org/stats_hip.html. Accessed February 2, 2017.

17. Banfield CM, Bartels JE, Hudson JA, et al. A retrospective study of canine hip dysplasia in 116 military working dogs. Part I: angle measurements and Orthopedic Foundation for Animals (OFA) grading. J Am Anim Hosp Assoc 1996;32:413–22.

18. Tsai KL, Murphy KE. Clinical and genetic assessments of hip joint laxity in the Boykin spaniel. Can J Vet Res 2006;70:148–50.

19. Gatineau M, Dupuis J, Beauregard G, et al. Palpation and dorsal acetabular rim radiographic projection for early detection of canine hip dysplasia: a prospective study. Vet Surg 2012;41:42–53.

20. Lust G, Williams AJ, Burton-Wurster N, et al. Joint laxity and its association with hip dysplasia in Labrador retrievers. Am J Vet Res 1993;54:1990–9.

21. Hays L, Zhang Z, Mateescu RG, et al. Quantitative genetics of secondary hip joint osteoarthritis in a Labrador retriever-greyhound pedigree. Am J Vet Res 2007;68: 35–41.

22. Ginja MMD, Ferreira AJ, Jesus SS, et al. Comparison of clinical, radiographic, computed tomographic, and magnetic resonance imaging methods for early prediction of canine hip laxity and dysplasia. Vet Radiol Ultrasound 2009;50:135–43.

23. Madsen JS. The joint capsule and joint laxity in dogs with hip dysplasia. J Am Vet Med Assoc 1997;210:1463–5.

24. Runge JJ, Kelly SP, Gregor TP, et al. Distraction index as a risk factor for osteoarthritis associated with hip dysplasia in four large dog breeds. J Small Anim Pract 2010;51:264–9.

25. Olsewski JM, Lust G, Rending VT, et al. Degenerative joint disease: multiple joint involvement in young and mature dogs. Am J Vet Res 1983;44:1300–8.

26. Farquhar T, Bertram J, Todhunter RJ, et al. Variations in composition of cartilage from the shoulder joints of young adult dogs at risk for developing canine hip dysplasia. J Am Vet Med Assoc 1997;210:1483–5.

27. Riser WH. The dysplastic hip joint: radiologic and histologic development. Vet Pathol 1975;12:279–305.

28. Smith GK, Gregor TP, Rhodes WH, et al. Coxofemoral joint laxity from distraction radiography and its contemporaneous and prospective correlation with laxity, subjective score, and evidence of degenerative joint disease from conventional hip-extended radiography in dogs. Am J Vet Res 1993;54:1021–42.

29. Evans HE. Miller's anatomy of the dog. 3rd edition. Philadelphia: WB Saunders; 1993. p. 349.

30. Lust G, Bellman WT, Rending VT. A relationship between degree of laxity and synovial fluid volume in coxofemoral joints of dogs predisposed for hip dysplasia. Am J Vet Res 1980;41:55–60.

31. Innes JF. Arthritis. In: Tobias KM, Johnston SA, editors. Veterinary surgery small animal, vol. 1, 1st edition. St Louis (MO): Elsevier; 2012. p. 1078–111.
32. Smith GK, LaFond E, Heyman SJ, et al. Biomechanical characterization of passive laxity of the hip joint in dogs. Am J Vet Res 1997;58:1078–82.
33. Madsen JS, Oxlund H, Svalastoga E, et al. Collagen type III: I composition in hip joints of dogs susceptible to hip dysplasia. J Small Anim Pract 1994;35:625–8.
34. Todhunter RJ, Zaches TA, Gilbert RO, et al. Onset of epiphyseal mineralization and growth plate closure in radiographically normal and dysplastic Labrador retrievers. J Am Vet Med Assoc 1997;210:1458–62.
35. Komsta R, Łojszczyk-Szczepaniak A, Dębiak P. Lumbosacral transitional vertebrae, canine hip dysplasia, and sacroiliac joint degenerative changes on ventrodorsal radiographs of the pelvis in police working German shepherd dogs. Top Companion Anim Med 2015;30:10–5.
36. D'Amico LL, Xie L, Abell LK, et al. Relationships of hip joint volume ratios with degrees of joint laxity and degenerative disease from youth to maturity in a canine population predisposed to hip joint osteoarthritis. Am J Vet Res 2011;72:376–83.
37. Smith GK, Lawler DF, Biery DN, et al. Chronology of hip dysplasia development in a cohort of 48 Labrador retrievers followed for life. Vet Surg 2012;41:20–33.
38. Alexander JW. The pathogenesis of canine hip dysplasia. Vet Clin North Am Small Anim Pract 1992;22:503–11.
39. Gold RM, Gregor TP, Huck JL, et al. Effects of osteoarthritis on radiographic measures of laxity and congruence in hip joints of Labrador Retrievers. J Am Vet Med Assoc 2009;234:1549–54.
40. Steffey MA, Todhunter RJ. Osteoarthritis. In: Bojrab MJ, Monnet E, editors. Mechanisms of disease in small animal surgery. 3rd edition. Jackson (WY): Teton NewMedia; 2010. p. 731–42.
41. Fujita Y, Hara Y, Nezu Y, et al. Direct and indirect markers of cartilage metabolism in synovial fluid obtained from dogs with hip dysplasia and correlation with clinical and radiographic variables. Am J Vet Res 2005;66:2028–33.
42. Chalmers HJ, Dykes NL, Lust G, et al. Assessment of bone mineral density of the femoral head in dogs with early osteoarthritis. Am J Vet Res 2006;67:796–800.
43. Lewis TW, Blott SC, Woolliams JA. Comparative analyses of genetic trends and prospects for selection against hip and elbow dysplasia in 15 UK dog breeds. BMC Genet 2013;14:16.
44. Leighton EA. Genetics of canine hip dysplasia. J Am Vet Med Assoc 1997;210: 1474–9.
45. van Hagen M, Ducro B, Broek J. Incidence, risk factors, and heritability estimates of hind limb lameness caused by hip dysplasia in a birth cohort of boxers. Am J Vet Res 2005;66:307–12.
46. Wood JLN, Lakhani KH, Rogers K. Heritability and epidemiology of canine hipdysplasia score and its components in Labrador retrievers in the United Kingdom. Prev Vet Med 2002;55:95–108.
47. Reed A, Keller G, Vogt D. Effect of dam and sire qualitative hip conformation scores on progeny hip conformation. J Am Vet Med Assoc 2000;217:675–80.
48. Zhang Z, Zhu L, Sandler J, et al. Estimation of heritabilities, genetic correlations, and breeding values of four traits that collectively define hip dysplasia in dogs. Am J Vet Res 2009;70:483–92.
49. Leppänen M, Mäki K, Juga J, et al. Factors affecting hip dysplasia in German shepherd dogs in Finland: efficacy of the current improvement programme. J Small Anim Pract 2000;41:19.

50. Willis MB. A review of the progress in canine hip dysplasia control in Britain. J Am Vet Med Assoc 1997;210:1480–2.

51. Kaneene JB, Mostosky UV, Miller R. Update of a retrospective cohort study of changes in hip joint phenotype of dogs evaluated by the OFA in the United States, 1989–2003. Vet Surg 2009;38:398–405.

52. Hou Y, Wang Y, Lust G, et al. Retrospective analysis for genetic improvement of hip joints of cohort Labrador retrievers in the United States: 1970–2007. PLoS One 2010;5:e9410.

53. Wilson BJ, Nicholas FW, James JW, et al. Genetic correlations among canine hip dysplasia radiographic traits in a cohort of Australian German shepherd dogs, and implications for the design of a more effective genetic control program. PLoS One 2013;8:e78929.

54. Bliss S, Todhunter RJ, Quaas R, et al. Quantitative genetics of traits associated with hip dysplasia in a canine pedigree constructed by mating dysplastic Labrador retrievers with unaffected greyhounds. Am J Vet Res 2002;63:1029–35.

55. Zhu L, Zhang Z, Friedenberg S, et al. The long (and winding) road to gene discovery for canine hip dysplasia. Vet J 2009;181:97–110.

56. Verhoeven G, Fortrie R, van Ryssen B, et al. Worldwide screening for canine hip dysplasia: where are we now? Vet Surg 2012;41:10–9.

57. Marschall Y, Distl O. Mapping quantitative trait loci for canine hip dysplasia in German shepherd dogs. Mamm Genome 2007;18:861–70.

58. Todhunter RJ, Mateescu R, Lust G, et al. Quantitative trait loci for hip dysplasia in a cross-breed canine pedigree. Mamm Genome 2005;16:720–30.

59. Phavaphutanon J, Mateescu RG, Tsai KL, et al. Evaluation of quantitative trait loci for hip dysplasia in Labrador retrievers. Am J Vet Res 2009;70:1094–101.

60. Chase K, Lawler DF, Carrier DR, et al. Genetic regulation of osteoarthritis: a QTL regulating cranial and caudal acetabular osteophyte formation in the hip joint of the dog (Canis familiaris). Am J Med Genet A 2005;135:334–5.

61. Friedenberg SG, Zhu L, Zhang Z, et al. Evaluation of a fibrillin 2 gene haplotype associated with hip dysplasia and incipient osteoarthritis in dogs. Am J Vet Res 2011;72:530–40.

62. Sánchez-Molano E, Woolliams JA, Pong-Wong R, et al. Quantitative trait loci mapping for canine hip dysplasia and its related traits in UK Labrador retrievers. BMC Genomics 2014;15:833.

63. Guo G, Zhou Z, Wang Y, et al. Canine hip dysplasia is predictable by genotyping. Osteoarthritis Cartilage 2011;19:420–9.

64. Bartolomé N, Segarra S, Artieda M, et al. A genetic predictive model for canine hip dysplasia: Integration of Genome Wide Association Study (GWAS) and candidate gene approaches. PLoS One 2015;10:e0122558.

65. Kealy RD, Olsson SE, Monti KL, et al. Effects of limited food consumption on the incidence of hip dysplasia in growing dogs. J Am Vet Med Assoc 1992;201: 857–63.

66. Kealy RD, Lawler DF, Ballam JM, et al. Five-year longitudinal study on limited food consumption and development of osteoarthritis in coxofemoral joints of dogs. J Am Vet Med Assoc 1997;210:222–5.

67. Kealy RD, Lawler DF, Ballam JM, et al. Evaluation of the effect of limited food consumption on radiographic evidence of osteoarthritis in dogs. J Am Vet Med Assoc 2000;217:1678–80.

68. Krontveit RI, Nødtvedt A, Sævik BK, et al. A prospective study on canine hip dysplasia and growth in a cohort of four large breeds in Norway (1998–2001). Prev Vet Med 2010;97:252–63.

69. Lopez MJ, Quinn MM, Markel MD. Associations between canine juvenile weight gain and coxofemoral joint laxity at 16 weeks of age. Vet Surg 2006;35:214–8.
70. Madsen JS, Reimann I, Svalastoga E. Delayed ossification of the femoral head in dogs with hip dysplasia. J Small Anim Pract 1991;32:351.
71. Kealy RD, Lawler DF, Monti KL, et al. Effects of dietary electrolyte balance on subluxation of the femoral head in growing dogs. Am J Vet Res 1993;54:555–62.
72. Riser WH, Shirer JF. Correlation between canine hip dysplasia and pelvic muscle mass: a study of 95 dogs. Am J Vet Res 1967;28:769–77.
73. Steinetz BG, Goldsmith LT, Lust G. Plasma relaxin levels in pregnant and lactating dogs. Biol Reprod 1987;37:719.
74. Lust G, Williams AJ, Burton-Wurster N, et al. Effects of intramuscular administration of glycosaminoglycan polysulfates on signs of incipient hip dysplasia in growing pups. Am J Vet Res 1992;53:1836–43.
75. Rettenmaier JL, Keller GG, Lattimer JC, et al. Prevalence of canine hip dysplasia in a veterinary teaching hospital population. Vet Radiol Ultrasound 2002;43: 313–8.
76. Witsberger TH, Villamil JA, Schultz LG, et al. Prevalence of and risk factors for hip dysplasia and cranial cruciate ligament deficiency in dogs. J Am Vet Med Assoc 2008;232:1818–24.
77. Paster ER, LaFond E, Biery DN, et al. Estimates of prevalence of hip dysplasia in golden retrievers and rottweilers and the influence of bias on published prevalence figures. J Am Vet Med Assoc 2005;226:387–92.
78. Powers MY, Karbe GT, Gregor TP, et al. Evaluation of the relationship between Orthopedic Foundation for Animals' hip joint scores and PennHIP distraction index values in dogs. J Am Vet Med Assoc 2010;237:532–41.
79. LaFond E, Breur GJ, Austin CC. Breed susceptibility for developmental orthopedic diseases in dogs. J Am Anim Hosp Assoc 2002;38:467–77.

Hip Dysplasia
Clinical Signs and Physical Examination Findings

Jason Syrcle, DVM

KEYWORDS

- Hip dysplasia • Hip laxity • Hip subluxation • Hip osteoarthritis • Ortolani test

KEY POINTS

- Hip dysplasia is a common developmental disorder of the dog consisting of varying degrees of hip laxity, progressive remodeling of the structures of the hip, and subsequent development of osteoarthritis.
- Hip dysplasia is a juvenile-onset condition, with clinical signs often first evident at 4 to 12 months of age.
- A presumptive diagnosis of hip dysplasia can be made by collection of a thorough history and performance of a comprehensive physical examination.
- The Ortolani test is a valuable screening tool for hip dysplasia, particularly in the juvenile patient.

INTRODUCTION

Hip dysplasia is a common developmental disorder of the dog, consisting of varying degrees of hip laxity, progressive remodeling of the structures of the hip, and subsequent development of osteoarthritis. Hip dysplasia may initially be suspected from signalment, history, and physical examination findings. This article outlines the typical clinical presentation of hip dysplasia and physical examination methods that can be used to help diagnose the condition and rule out other problems.

SIGNALMENT
Breed

Any size or breed of dog can be affected with hip dysplasia but the condition is most commonly diagnosed in large and giant breed dogs. Breeds with the most evaluations by the Orthopedic Foundation for Animals for hip dysplasia over the last 40 years

The author has nothing to disclose.
Small Animal Surgery, Department of Clinical Sciences, College of Veterinary Medicine, Mississippi State University, PO Box 6100, Mississippi State, MS 39762, USA
E-mail address: syrcle@cvm.msstate.edu

include Labrador Retrievers (12.2% dysplastic), Golden Retrievers (20.1%), German Shepherds (20.4%), and Rottweilers (21.3%). Breeds with particularly high reported prevalence of dysplasia include the Bulldog (73.4%), Pug (69.7%), and St. Bernard (49.2%).[1] These numbers do not indicate a true prevalence because breeders typically will not submit radiographs from dogs that are obviously dysplastic. Although certain dog breeds are predisposed, mixed-breed dogs can also develop hip dysplasia. In one large study, purebreds and mixed-breed dogs were equally likely to develop hip dysplasia.[2]

Sex

Multiple large prevalence studies show no sex predilection associated with hip dysplasia.[3–6] However, several studies suggest that male neutered dogs may be at increased risk for development of hip dysplasia, especially when neutered early.[7–10] Definitions of early neutering associated with increased incidence of hip dysplasia in these studies included dogs that were younger than 5.5 months, 6 months, and 12 months of age at the time of neutering.

Age

Juvenile patients

Hip dysplasia is by definition a juvenile-onset condition. Clinical signs of hip dysplasia are often first evident at 4 to 12 months of age.[11–13] Onset of signs is typically gradual and progressive, although an acute onset of signs may be seen, most often in juvenile patients. Dogs with this acute onset of signs are typically more severely affected, with pain thought to be caused by stretching and tearing of joint capsule and other supporting structures, along with acetabular microfracture.[13] Evidence of hip laxity is not present at birth but may be detectable as early as 7 weeks of age.[11] Clinical signs noted by the owner are listed in **Table 1**.[11–14]

Adult patients

Several reasons may exist for initial presentation of dysplastic patients older than 12 months of age. The patient may have had signs as a puppy that went unnoticed by the owner, undiagnosed by the family veterinarian, or there was a delay in referral. Alternatively, some dogs may not exhibit clinical signs until later in the disease process, often associated with progression of osteoarthritis. These cases may exhibit clinical signs similar to juvenile patients but clinical signs in older patients are often

Table 1 Clinical signs of hip dysplasia		
Nonspecific Signs	**Hind Limb Specific Signs**	**Gait Abnormalities**
• Exercise intolerance • Reluctance to navigate stairs • Difficulty lying down or rising	• Audible click or clunk when walking • Perceived hip pain • Hind limb muscle atrophy • Unilateral hind limb lameness	• Hind end sways when walking • Wobbly or ataxic-appearing gait, with normal neurologic examination • Walking with an arched back • Base-narrow or base-wide stance of the hind limbs • Bunny hopping

more referable to osteoarthritic changes, rather than signs associated with laxity and subluxation. Because clinical signs of hip dysplasia in older patients are most often gradually progressive, an adult patient presenting for acute onset of hind limb lameness attributed to hip dysplasia should be carefully screened for other conditions.

PHYSICAL EXAMINATION FINDINGS
Lameness Evaluation

Any of the gait abnormalities referenced in **Table 1** can be seen on examination. Although hip dysplasia is typically a bilateral condition, sometimes clinical signs are more severe on one side and a unilateral lameness may be appreciated.

Orthopedic Examination

Systematic orthopedic examination should localize discomfort to the hips. For dysplastic patients, hip manipulation is typically painful, particularly hip extension. Pain on hip extension should be differentiated from other conditions. Common differential diagnoses for pain localized to the hip are listed in **Table 2**. In addition to hip pain, patients with advanced osteoarthritis may also exhibit crepitus on palpation of the hip, as well as decreased coxofemoral range-of motion and muscle atrophy of the affected limb. Complete orthopedic evaluation is critical because comorbidities may be present that complicate treatment recommendations. For example, an adult dog presenting with acute-onset hind limb lameness may indeed have hip dysplasia but the lameness may be attributable to a cranial cruciate ligament rupture.

Joint Subluxation Tests
Overview

Hip laxity can be identified and quantified by several examination methods, including the tests of Barlow, Ortolani, and Bardens.[15–17] The Ortolani and Barlow tests were developed for screening of hip dysplasia in infants. The positive Ortolani test involves abducting a subluxated hip until palpable and/or audible reduction of the hip is noted. This sensation is often described as a click or a clunk. The test can be performed in lateral or dorsal recumbency in the dog. The Barlow test involves active subluxation of the hip. For this test, the hip is adducted while applying a distoproximal force. The subluxation can be sensed as an acute proximal displacement of the hip with palpable loss of stability. This can also be performed in dorsal or lateral recumbency. The Bardens test, described by a veterinarian in the late 1960s, involves applying a mediolateral force to the proximal femur with 1 hand while quantifying lateral movement of the greater trochanter with the other. This test is performed in lateral recumbency. Any palpable reduction or subluxation with the Ortolani or Barlow test, or lateral movement of the greater trochanter of more than about 6 mm with the Bardens test, should be considered abnormal and evidence of hip laxity.

Table 2	
Common differential diagnoses for dogs with hip pain and no history of trauma	
Juvenile	**Adult**
• Iliopsoas strain	• Iliopsoas strain
• Legg-Calvé-Perthes disease (small breeds)	• Lumbosacral stenosis
• Slipped capital femoral physis	• Neoplasia

Ortolani test

The author's preference when assessing hip subluxation in juvenile patients is to perform a combination of the Barlow and Ortolani tests (commonly referred to as an Ortolani test), as described by Chalman and Butler[18] in 1985. The patient is heavily sedated or anesthetized and placed in dorsal recumbency. An assistant stabilizes the thorax and head of the dog to ensure true dorsal recumbency is maintained. The examiner is behind the patient, looking toward the head. The examiner grasps the stifles and ensures the femurs are positioned perpendicular to the floor (**Fig. 1**). Each hip is tested sequentially, as follows. Gentle pressure is applied down the shaft of the femur toward the acetabulum (**Fig. 2A**). While maintaining this downward pressure, the hip is slowly abducted until a palpable clunk is noted. The angle of the medial aspect of the femur with a line perpendicular to the examination table is noted at the time of reduction of the hip and recorded as the angle of reduction (see **Fig. 2B**). If no palpable or audible reduction of the hip is noted, this is a negative Ortolani test result. The hip is then adducted until subluxation is noted, palpable as a dorsal deviation of the proximal femur. The angle of the medial aspect of the femur with a line perpendicular to the examination table is recorded as the angle of subluxation (see **Fig. 2C**). The test is often repeated 2 to 3 times for each hip to ensure accuracy and precision of the measurements. The reduction and subluxation angles, as well as the nature of the reduction (crisp or soft) are recorded. These data may be useful to quantify hip laxity, follow progression of changes over time and to judge candidacy for surgical interventions such as juvenile pubic symphysiodesis or triple pelvic osteotomy.

Evidence: Ortolani test

Dogs with a positive Ortolani test were associated with increasing distraction index (DI) measurements in a group of dogs in one study.[19] In that report, dogs were categorized as having a mild, moderate, or severe Ortolani sign, with mild being a barely perceptible reduction and severe being a loud or obvious clunk. Increasing DI was

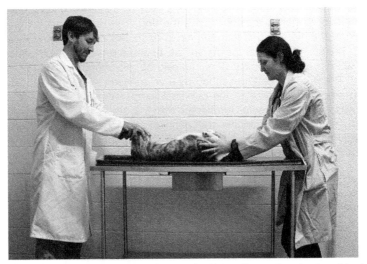

Fig. 1. Examination of a patient using the Ortolani test. The patient is placed in dorsal recumbency with an assistant to stabilize the thorax and head. The examiner stands behind the patient, grasping the stifles, with the femurs positioned perpendicular to the floor.

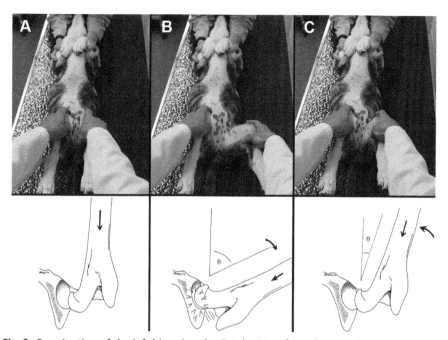

Fig. 2. Examination of the left hip using the Ortolani test from the examiner's perspective, paired with drawings depicting effects of the test on the coxofemoral joint. (*A*) Gentle pressure is applied down the shaft (*arrow*) of the left femur with the examiner's right hand, causing subluxation of the hip. (*B*) While maintaining this downward pressure (*arrow*), the hip is slowly abducted (*curved arrow*) until a palpable clunk is noted. The angle of the medial aspect of the femur with a line perpendicular to the examination table is measured at the time of reduction of the hip and recorded as the angle of reduction (angle θ). (*C*) The hip is adducted (*curved arrow*) while continuing to maintain downward pressure (*arrow*) until subluxation is noted, palpable as a dorsal deviation of the proximal femur. The angle of the medial aspect of the femur with a line perpendicular to the examination table is recorded as the angle of subluxation (angle θ).

associated with increasing severity of the Ortolani, suggesting increased laxity could be semiquantified with the test. The same study showed the association between DI and Ortolani was weaker in dogs with radiographic osteoarthritis, suggesting that remodeling in such cases led to a negative or decreased Ortolani sign, despite laxity of the hip. Ortolani testing has been shown to provide a 92% to 100% sensitivity for identifying laxity in juvenile dogs older than 4 months of age that later developed radiographic signs of hip dysplasia.[20–22] Specificity in those studies study was 41% to 79%, suggesting Ortolani evaluation might best be used as a screening test and other tests, such as DI measurements, may be better for confirmation of diagnosis. However, a study evaluating Ortolani in younger dogs (6–10 weeks of age) revealed a lower sensitivity for detecting dysplastic dogs (55%), so caution should be used when proclaiming a young puppy free of hip dysplasia using the Ortolani test alone.[23] Additionally, subluxation tests may become less productive as dysplasia progresses.[19] As dorsal acetabular rim wear and acetabular infilling increases in severity, reduction of the subluxated hip becomes less distinct or no longer palpable. Therefore, the Ortolani and other subluxation tests may be less valuable for evaluating older dogs with suspected hip dysplasia.

SUMMARY

With proper attention to collection of history and physical examination findings, the clinician can eliminate differential diagnoses and make a presumptive diagnosis of hip dysplasia. The Ortolani test is a valuable tool for identifying juvenile dogs affected with this condition. Further diagnostics can then be prioritized, contributing to prompt diagnosis and appropriate treatment.

ACKNOWLEDGMENTS

The author would like to thank Jonathan Blakely, DVM for providing the line drawings used in this article.

REFERENCES

1. Orthopedic Foundation for Animals. Hip Dysplasia Statistics. Available at: http://www.offa.org/stats_hip.html. Accessed June 9, 2016.
2. Bellumori TP, Famula TR, Bannasch DL, et al. Prevalence of inherited disorders among mixed-breed and purebred dogs: 27,254 cases (1995-2010). J Am Vet Med Assoc 2013;242:1549–55.
3. Hou Y, Wang Y, Lu X, et al. Monitoring hip and elbow dysplasia achieved modest genetic improvement of 74 dog breeds over 40 years in USA. PLoS One 2013;8: e76390.
4. Krontveit RI, Trangerud C, Nødtvedt A, et al. The effect of radiological hip dysplasia and breed on survival in a prospective cohort study of four large dog breeds followed over a 10 year period. Vet J 2012;193:206–11.
5. Runge JJ, Kelly SP, Gregor TP, et al. Distraction index as a risk factor for osteoarthritis associated with hip dysplasia in four large dog breeds. J Small Anim Pract 2010;51:264–9.
6. Hou Y, Wang Y, Lust G, et al. Retrospective analysis for genetic improvement of hip joints of cohort Labrador retrievers in the United States: 1970-2007. PLoS One 2010;5:e9410.
7. Witsberger TH, Villamil JA, Schultz LG, et al. Prevalence of and risk factors for hip dysplasia and cranial cruciate ligament deficiency in dogs. J Am Vet Med Assoc 2008;232:1818–24.
8. Torres de la Riva G, Hart BL, Farver TB, et al. Neutering dogs: effects on joint disorders and cancers in golden retrievers. PLoS One 2013;8:e55937.
9. van Hagen MA, Ducro BJ, van den Broek J, et al. Incidence, risk factors, and heritability estimates of hind limb lameness caused by hip dysplasia in a birth cohort of boxers. Am J Vet Res 2005;66:307–12.
10. Spain CV, Scarlett JM, Houpt KA. Long-term risks and benefits of early-age gonadectomy in dogs. J Am Vet Med Assoc 2004;224:380–7.
11. Riser WH, Rhodes WH, Newton CD. Hip dysplasia. In: Newton CD, Nunamaker DM, editors. Textbook of small animal orthopedics. Philadelphia: JB Lippincott; 1985. p. 953–80.
12. Wallace LJ, Olmstead ML. Disabling conditions of the coxofemoral joint. In: Olmstead ML, editor. Small animal orthopedics. St Louis (MO): Mosby; 1995. p. 361–93.
13. Piermattei DL, Flo GL, DeCamp CE. The hip joint. In: Piermattei DL, Flo GL, DeCamp CE, editors. Brinker, Piermattei, and Flo's handbook of small animal orthopedics and fracture repair. 4th edition. St Louis (MO): Saunders Elsevier; 2006. p. 416–511.

14. Slocum B, Slocum TD. Hip. In: Bojrab MJ, editor. Current techniques in small animal surgery. 4th edition. Baltimore (MD): Williams & Wilkins; 1998. p. 1127–85.
15. Barlow TG. Early diagnosis and treatment of congenital dislocation of the hip. Proc R Soc Med 1963;56:804–6.
16. Ortolani M. Congenital hip dysplasia in the light of early and very early diagnosis. Clin Orthop Relat Res 1976;119:6–10.
17. Bardens JW, Hardwick H. New observations on the diagnosis and cause of hip dysplasia. Vet Med Small Anim Clin 1968;63:238–45.
18. Chalman JA, Butler HC. Coxofemoral joint laxity and the Ortolani sign. J Am Anim Hosp Assoc 1985;21:671–6.
19. Puerto DA, Smith GK, Gregor TP, et al. Relationships between results of the Ortolani method of hip joint palpation and distraction index, Norberg angle, and hip score in dogs. J Am Vet Med Assoc 1999;214:497–501.
20. Ginja MM, Silvestre AM, Colaço J, et al. Hip dysplasia in Estrela mountain dogs: prevalence and genetic trends 1991-2005. Vet J 2009;182:275–82.
21. Gatineau M, Dupuis J, Beauregard G, et al. Palpation and dorsal acetabular rim radiographic projection for early detection of canine hip dysplasia: a prospective study. Vet Surg 2012;41:42–53.
22. Corfield GS, Read RA, Eastley KA, et al. Assessment of the hip reduction angle for predicting osteoarthritis of the hip in the Labrador retriever. Aust Vet J 2007; 85:212–6.
23. Adams WM, Dueland RT, Meinen J, et al. Early detection of canine hip dysplasia: comparison of two palpation and five radiographic methods. J Am Anim Hosp Assoc 1998;34:339–47.

Canine Hip Dysplasia
Diagnostic Imaging

J. Ryan Butler, DVM, MS[a],*, Jennifer Gambino, DVM[b]

KEYWORDS

- Hip-extended radiographs • Distraction radiography • Hip osteoarthritis
- Norberg angle • Computed tomography • MRI

KEY POINTS

- A properly positioned hip-extended radiograph is useful as a screening tool for hip dysplasia and for detection of osteoarthritis but may not adequately represent the degree of hip laxity.
- The caudal curvilinear osteophyte (Morgan line) and circumferential femoral head osteophyte represent 2 of the earliest signs of coxofemoral osteoarthritis.
- A PennHip distraction index of ≥ 0.3 in dogs ≥ 16 weeks of age is generally considered to indicate an increased risk of future osteoarthritis development.
- MRI modalities such as T2 mapping and dGEMRIC imaging allow for a more sensitive assessment of cartilage health.

INTRODUCTION

Imaging of the canine pelvis couple with physical exam findings are the principle methods used to screen for and diagnose canine hip dysplasia, especially when evaluating juvenile patients in the early course of the disease. Once the disease has progressed to a state of severe osteoarthritis, the ability to diagnose the condition becomes less complicated because the radiographic changes are more readily apparent. Many imaging modalities such as radiography, computed tomography (CT), ultrasound, and MRI can be used in the assessment of canine patients with hip dysplasia. These imaging modalities are used for the preliminary diagnosis of hip dysplasia as well as in the surveillance of disease progression and the evaluation of the success of treatment interventions. Each imaging modality has inherent

Disclosure Statement: The authors have nothing to disclose.
[a] Small Animal Surgery, Department of Clinical Sciences, College of Veterinary Medicine, Mississippi State University, PO Box 6100, Mississippi State, MS 39762, USA; [b] Diagnostic Imaging, Department of Clinical Sciences, College of Veterinary Medicine, Mississippi State University, PO Box 6100, Mississippi State, MS 39762, USA
* Corresponding author.
E-mail address: ryan.butler@msstate.edu

advantages, disadvantages, and limitations. This article discusses the various imaging modalities and their utility with regard to canine hip dysplasia.

RADIOGRAPHY

Hip dysplasia is defined as radiographic evidence of joint laxity or signs of osteoarthritis, with hip laxity being the primary risk factor for osteoarthritis development.[1] Radiographs have been used for diagnosing hip dysplasia since the condition was first reported in 1935.[2] Numerous radiographic projections can be used to evaluate and screen patients. The most commonly reported techniques include hip-extended radiography, Norberg angle, distraction-stress radiographs, and the dorsal acetabular rim (DAR) view.

Hip-Extended Radiography

The ventrodorsal, hip-extended radiograph is the most commonly used radiographic projection for evaluating canine hips. Proper positioning for this view often requires heavy sedation and/or general anesthesia and is achieved by placing the animal in dorsal recumbency, extending the hind limbs caudally, and slightly internally rotating the femurs. A properly positioned radiograph should include a symmetric pelvis, parallel and fully extended femurs, and patellas that are centered within the femoral trochlea (**Fig. 1**A).[3] This radiographic position is the one most often used by screening organizations such as the Orthopedic Foundation for Animals (OFA), Fédération Cynologique Internationale, and the British Veterinary Association/Kennel Club. Common

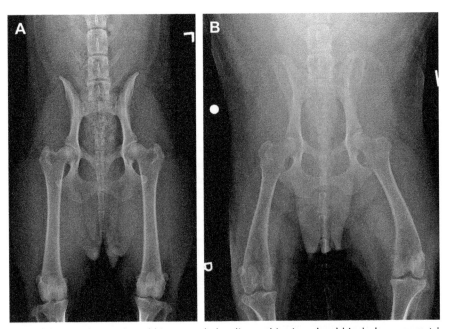

Fig. 1. (A) Properly positioned hip-extended radiographic view should include a symmetric pelvis, parallel and fully extended femurs, and patellas that are centered within the femoral trochlea. (B) Common errors in positioning include failure to fully extend and internally rotate the femurs.

errors in positioning include failure to fully extend the limbs and inadequate internal rotation of the femurs (**Fig. 1**B).

One of the main advantages of the hip-extended radiograph is the ability to evaluate the joint for signs of osteoarthritis. Radiographic evidence of osteoarthritis of the coxofemoral joint includes femoral periarticular osteophyte formation, subchondral sclerosis of the craniodorsal acetabulum, osteophytes along the acetabular margin, and joint remodeling (**Fig. 2**).[4] The caudal curvilinear osteophyte (CCO, or Morgan line) and circumferential femoral head osteophyte (CFHO) (**Fig. 3**) represent 2 radiographic

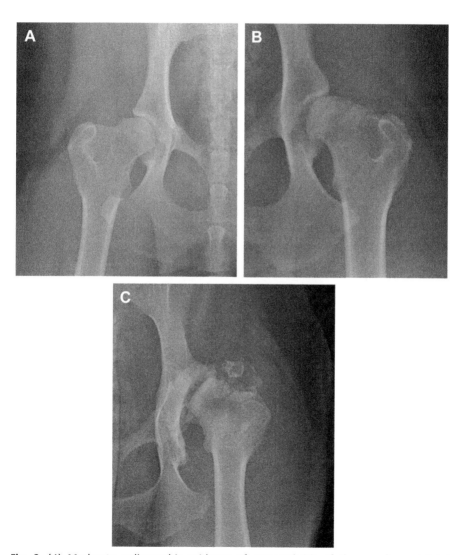

Fig. 2. (*A*) Moderate radiographic evidence of osteoarthritis of the coxofemoral joint including periarticular osteophyte formation and subchondral sclerosis of the craniodorsal acetabulum. (*B*) More severe cases include substantial thickening of the femoral neck. (*C*) Extreme cases can present with substantial joint remodeling and periarticular osteophytosis.

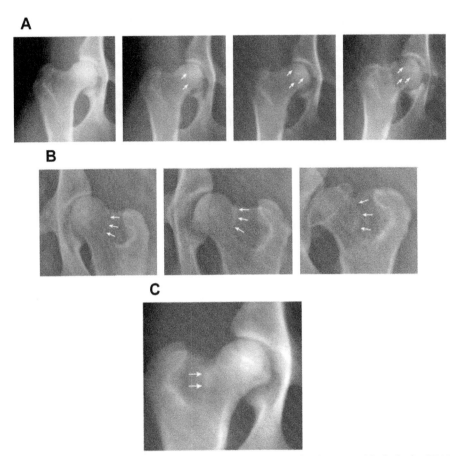

Fig. 3. Early radiographic signs of osteophytosis (as indicated by the *arrows*) include the CFHO (*A*) and the caudocurvilinear osteophyte (more specifically, an enthesophyte, also called a Morgan line) (*B*). Note the progression of periarticular osteophyte formation along the femoral neck and the increased opacity of the Morgan line. The puppy line (*arrows*) (*C*) is located in a similar location to the Morgan line and is typically seen in dogs less than 18 months of age. However, the puppy line is more diffuse and subtle when compared with the Morgan line and is of no clinical significance. (*From* Smith GK, Karba GT, Angello KA, et al. Pathogenesis, diagnosis, and control of canine hip dysplasia. In: Tobais KM, Johnson SA, editors. Veterinary surgery: small animal, vol. 1. 1st edition. St Louis (MO): Saunders/Elsevier; 2012. p. 836, with permission; and [*A*] Szabo SD, Biery DN, Lawler DF, et al. Evaluation of a circumferential femoral head osteophyte as an early indicator of osteoarthritis characteristic of canine hip dysplasia in dogs. J Am Vet Med Assoc 2007;231(6):890, with permission.)

features that have been reported to represent early osteophyte formation that predict later development of more characteristic signs of osteoarthritis.[5–9] However, the CCO and CFHO radiographic signs are not yet adopted by the screening organizations. The puppy line is a more subtle opacification of the femoral neck seen in the area of the CCO in young dogs (see **Fig. 3**C).[5,7,8] It is important to differentiate between the puppy line and the CCO because the puppy line represents an incidental finding that is often gone by 18 months of age and has no correlation with later development of osteoarthritis.[8]

Although radiographic evidence of osteoarthritis occurs in most cases of hip dysplasia, this clinical feature occurs later in the disease process.[3,10] In the absence of radiographic signs of osteoarthritis, joint subluxation on the hip-extended radiograph is considered diagnostic for hip dysplasia (**Fig. 4**).[11,12] The degree of subluxation can be subjectively evaluated or objectively quantified using methods such as the Norberg angle and femoral overlap (% coverage), which are discussed separately. However, the hip-extended radiograph may mask joint subluxation by tightening the joint capsule as the limbs are extended and forcing the femoral heads to sit more deeply with the acetabula. The joint capsule tightening can make dysplastic hips appear normal and may be a factor contributing to a high rate of false-negative radiographic evaluations.[13,14]

The relatively low interobserver and intraobserver agreement seen when used as a screening tool further complicates the incidence of false negative evaluations.[3,15–17] Even when specific radiographic markers of osteoarthritis such as the CFHO and CCO are evaluated, the reliability within and between experienced observers is low, which increases errors in the screening process and surgical decision making.[18]

Norberg Angle and Femoral Overlap

The Norberg angle and femoral overlap (otherwise known as % coverage) represent 2 means to objectively quantify the degree of femoral subluxation seen on hip-extended radiographs. The Norberg angle is calculated by measuring the angle between a line that connects the center of the femoral head between the left and right hips and a line

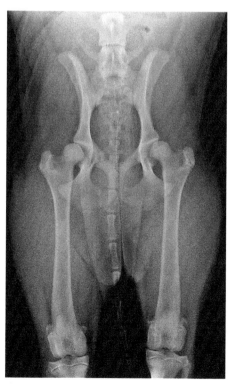

Fig. 4. Hip-extended radiograph of an immature dog with bilateral joint subluxation consistent with a diagnosis of hip dysplasia.

that connects the center of the femoral head with the lateral tip of the cranial acetabular rim **(Fig. 5A)**.[11] A larger angle indicates a deeper acetabulum and more congruent hips, whereas smaller angles are consistent with increasing degrees of subluxation. A Norberg angle of greater than 105° is generally considered to be normal.[19] Norberg angles less than 105° are consistent with hip laxity. Femoral overlap is also a measurement of femoral displacement from the acetabulum. Normal joint overlap is considered to be ≥50% with values less than this being consistent with joint incongruity **(Fig. 5B)**.[20] The percentage of femoral overlap is commonly used to determine the postoperative success of the triple pelvic osteotomy (TPO) procedure.[21]

Disadvantages of using either the Norberg angle or percentage of femoral overlap include the significant effect of pelvic positioning on the measurement and, as previously discussed, the possible effect of hip extension on joint laxity.[22] Slight rotation of the pelvis on the radiograph will substantially affect both the Norberg angle and the femoral overlap, causing the congruency of one hip joint to be overestimated, with underestimation of the contralateral hip joint.[22] Furthermore, the use of a strict reference value for the Norberg angle is not appropriate because a value consistent with dysplastic hips can vary between breeds.[23]

Distraction-Stress Radiographs

Distraction-stress radiography techniques are used to better estimate the degree of passive laxity of the coxofemoral articulation. Ideally, the techniques would determine the degree of laxity present during ambulation, otherwise known as functional laxity. However, a method that accurately determines functional laxity is not currently

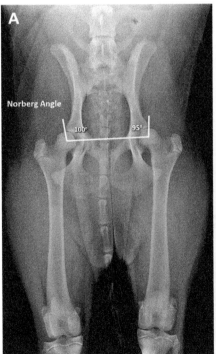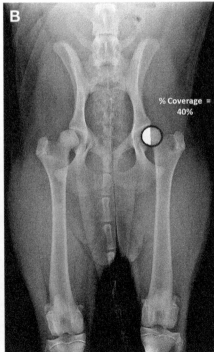

Fig. 5. Joint subluxation can be quantified with either the Norberg angle (*A*) or % Femoral Overlap (% Coverage) (*B*).

available. The distraction stress radiography methods most commonly used include the University of Pennsylvania Hip Improvement Program (PennHip), Dorsolateral Subluxation Measurement (DLS), and the Flückiger Subluxation Index.[20]

The PennHip method of radiography is performed in a heavily sedated or anesthetized animal. Three radiographic projections are obtained: a standard hip-extended radiograph, a neutral stance-phase compression radiograph, and a neutral stance-phase distraction radiograph (**Fig. 6**).[14] For the distraction radiograph, an acrylic fulcrum device is placed between the proximal femurs, and an adduction force results in hip subluxation in abnormal dogs. From the distraction radiograph, a distraction index (DI) can be calculated as the degree of femoral head subluxation from the

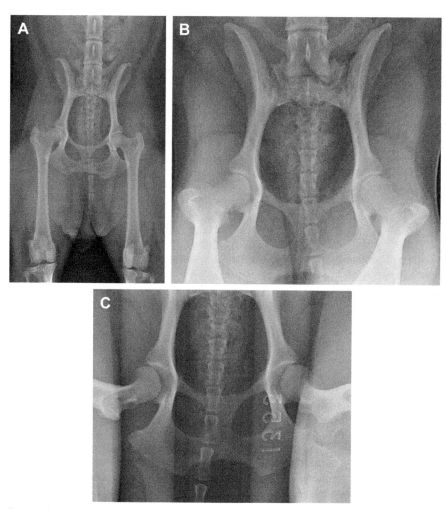

Fig. 6. The PennHip radiographic method includes 3 radiographic views: standard hip-extended radiograph (*A*), compression radiograph (*B*), and a distraction radiograph (*C*). The hip-extended radiograph is used to evaluate the joint for signs of osteoarthrosis; the compression radiograph is used to determine joint congruency (compression index), and the distraction radiograph is used to determine the degree of passive laxity (DI).

acetabulum. A DI score of 0 equates to no subluxation, whereas a DI score of 1 equates to a fully luxated joint.[20] The compression radiograph is used to evaluate joint congruency, as inability to fully compress the joints and achieve complete congruity (a compression index ≥ 0) may be an early estimator of osteoarthritis.[24] The hip-extended radiograph is used to evaluate the coxofemoral joints for standard evidence of osteoarthritis.

The significance of the DI score has been thoroughly investigated, and its significance in predicting the future development of osteoarthritis is reported.[5,25–28] A major advantage to the PennHip method is its ability to predict the future development of osteoarthritis in younger animals. The method can be predictive for osteoarthritis development in animals as young as 16 weeks of age.[27,29,30] In addition, the PennHip method allows researchers the ability to develop breed-specific DI profiles to provide a better estimate of future breed-related osteoarthritis development.[26,28] Although there are breed differences, a DI of greater than 0.3 is generally accepted as the cutoff value for osteoarthritis susceptibility.[31] However, the passive laxity measured by DI may not fully account for all forces acting across the joint in the awake and ambulatory dog. For example, a heavily muscled dog may be more tolerant of a higher DI and be less likely to develop osteoarthritis compared with a more petite dog of the same breed with the same DI.[32]

Because of its ability to predict osteoarthritis development at an earlier age, the PennHip method is often used for screening at-risk breeds before use for breeding, to determine candidacy for preventative procedures such as the juvenile pelvic symphysiodesis, or to initiate preventative measures such as calorie restriction in "at-risk" animals.[33,34] A minor disadvantage to the PennHip method is the requirement for veterinarians to attend a training course for certification in order to take and submit the radiographs. Although this likely improves the quality of film submission and the clinical relevance of the interpretations, it limits the availability of the program. It is important to note that the PennHip program is not a pass/fail or certifying program: it is a continuous scale that provides owners, breeders, and veterinarians information regarding the susceptibility of a patient for osteoarthritis development. However, definitive radiographic evidence of osteoarthritis will result in a designation of "confirmed hip dysplasia."[20]

The DLS is a distraction stress radiography technique that is similar in principle to the PennHip method, but less rigorously investigated. Positioning for the test aims to better simulate a weight-bearing position with the unrealistic goal of better estimating functional laxity. To perform the test, the animal is anesthetized and placed in sternal recumbency in a foam rubber mold with the hips flexed to a weight-bearing angle, femurs adducted, and the stifles flexed (**Fig. 7**).[20] In this position, the femurs are forced to dorsolaterally subluxate, and the degree of subluxation is quantified by determining the percentage of femoral overlap. A DLS score of 56% has been reported to have similar clinical implications as a DI score of greater than 0.3.[27,35,36] However, long-term studies in large populations of dogs are lacking. Furthermore, as with the hip-extended method of radiography, the DLS score is highly dependent on proper patient positioning and can be affected by arthritic changes within the joint.[20] Opponents of the technique also argue that the method does not truly place the animal in a weight-bearing position because the hips are actually more extended and adducted.[20] Because of the lack of long-term studies and issues associated with patient positioning, the clinical utility of this method is questionable.

The Flückiger Subluxation Index is similar in principle to the DLS method. However, the animals are placed in dorsal recumbency with a lesser degree of hip adduction (**Fig. 8**).[37] A dorsally directed force is applied to the limbs, which results in dorsolateral

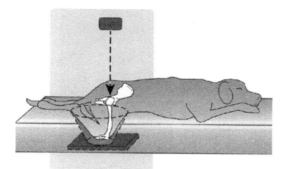

Fig. 7. To position a dog for the dorsolateral subluxation radiographic view, the patient is placed in a rubber mold with the limbs adducted and the distal femurs slightly caudal to the greater trochanters. (*From* Smith GK, Karba GT, Angello KA, et al. Pathogenesis, diagnosis, and control of canine hip dysplasia. In: Tobais KM, Johnson SA, editors. Veterinary surgery: small animal, vol. 1. 1st edition. St Louis (MO): Saunders/Elsevier; 2012. p. 840; with permission.)

hip subluxation. From the radiographs, circular gauges are placed over the femoral heads and acetabula for calculation of a subluxation index, which is similar to the DI. No studies have been performed that report the sensitivity, specificity, or predictability for osteoarthritis development for this diagnostic method.[20]

Dorsal Acetabular Rim View

The DAR view was first described by Slocum and Devine[38] in 1990. This radiographic view is used to evaluate the dorsal aspect of the acetabular rim, which is the area of the acetabulum that receives much of the stress concentration with subluxation of the femoral head during ambulation.[12,39–41] The DAR view achieves an unobstructed view of the dorsal acetabula from a cranial to caudal perspective. To obtain this radiograph, the patient is anesthetized and placed in sternal recumbency, and the rear limbs are pulled cranially and held close to the animal's body (**Fig. 9**). A spacer can be placed below the tarsi to provide additional pelvic rotation. Correct radiographic positioning results in superimposition of the iliac wings, iliac body, acetabulum, and tuber ischii, with an unobstructed view of the dorsal acetabula.[38]

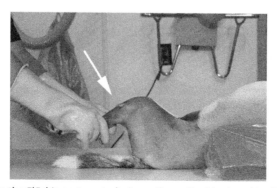

Fig. 8. To perform the Flückiger stress technique, the patient is placed in dorsal recumbency with the hips extended to approximately 60° from the table top. A dorsally directed force (*arrow*) results in coxofemoral subluxation in dysplastic dogs. The laxity is quantified radiographically in manner similar to the PennHip radiographic method.

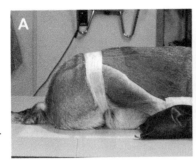
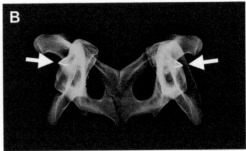

Fig. 9. To position for the DAR view (*A*), the patient is placed in sternal recumbency with the hind limbs pulled forward. The limbs are held parallel with the body with tape and the tarsi are slightly elevated with sandbags. (*B*) This view allows visualization of the DARs (*arrows, outlined in yellow*) as demonstrated in this pelvis model.

The DAR view is reportedly useful to document the degree of joint damage as the acetabular rim progresses from sharply pointed in the normal dog to more rounded and blunted with joint damage.[42] However, the portion of the acetabula evaluated by the DAR view, the DAR point, has been shown be approximately 37° caudal to the point of maximum wear in the standing animal and may underrepresent changes to the DAR.[43] Some surgeons also use this view to measure the dorsal acetabular slope to determine the appropriate degree of pelvic rotation when performing a TPO.[38,42,44–47] However, the DAR radiographic view is not widely used because diagnostic quality images can be difficult to obtain, and there is limited clinical utility of the study when compared with other diagnostic methods such as joint palpation or DI calculations.[32]

ULTRASOUND

Ultrasound imaging of human neonates has been used since 1980 as a screening tool for hip dysplasia in at-risk patients.[48,49] A similar technique has also been described in the dog to detect joint laxity with mixed results.[50–53] Disadvantages of the technique include inability to evaluate acetabular morphology after approximately 8 weeks of age in dogs because of femoral head ossification, subjectivity of the evaluation and scoring systems, and the lack of normal reference values.[20]

Ultrasound of the canine hip usually includes a subjective assessment of the acetabular morphology, determination of the acetabular angle of inclination (α-angle), and cartilage roof angle (β-angle). The α-angle is an indicator of the bony remodeling of the acetabulum, and the β-angle is an indicator of acetabular cartilage remodeling **(Fig. 10)**. Dynamic sonographic techniques also attempt to determine joint laxity by reporting a distraction value.[51] Generally, lower α-angle values are consistent with a shallow acetabulum, and higher β-angles are consistent with blunting of the cartilage rim.[50–53] However, these ultrasonographic variables in young animals had no correlation with the diagnosis of hip dysplasia in the mature animals.[51] Furthermore, the clinical utility of the ultrasound is highly operator dependent. For these reasons, ultrasound is not routinely used for diagnosing or screening canine patients for hip dysplasia.[20]

COMPUTED TOMOGRAPHY

CT, although becoming more readily available in veterinary medicine, is not used routinely for the evaluation of canine hips and is seldom used in pediatric patients

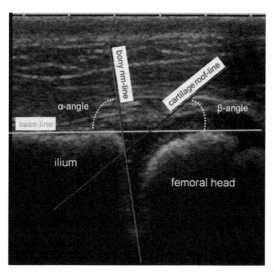

Fig. 10. Ultrasonographic measurement of hip congruity. The baseline (*green*) is parallel with the ilial silhouette. The bony rimline (*red*) is drawn connecting the caudal edge of the ilium in the acetabular fossa to the osseous convexity of the acetabular rim. The cartilage roof-line (*blue*) connects the osseous convexity of the bony acetabular rim to the cartilage roof triangle. The α-angle is the angle between the baseline and bony rimline. The β-angle is the angle between the cartilage roof-line and the baseline. (*From* Fischer A, Flöck A, Tellhelm B, et al. Static and dynamic ultrasonography for the early diagnosis of canine hip dysplasia. J Small Anim Pract 2010;51:582; with permission.)

due to risks associated with ionizing radiation. Historically, the use of this modality in people, and in canine research, supports the theory that the modality has merit in the evaluation of dysplastic changes.[20] CT provides accurate and easy evaluation of coxofemoral joint indices while the animal is positioned in a weight-bearing position, which may be a better indicator of the degree of functional laxity.[54] Various CT hip indices have been compared with PennHip and OFA conformation scores in an attempt to predict hip microdamage and correlate findings with those seen on the PennHip and OFA evaluations. Both the center edge angle (CEA) and dorsal acetabular sector angle (DASA) were shown to correlate with the PennHip DI and joint microdamage at 30 months of age in a cohort of research dogs predisposed to coxofemoral osteoarthritis (**Fig. 11**).[55] Furthermore, the combined measures of CEA and DI and the combined measures of DASA and Norberg Angle at 16 and 32 weeks of age, respectively, were found to be predictive of future osteoarthritis development in the mature animal.[56] However, the normal reference ranges for these CT values and the ability of these values to predict joint microdamage in a heterogeneous population of dogs requires further investigation.

MRI

Conventional MRI is infrequently used for the evaluation of canine developmental bone disorders in general. As an imaging modality, MRI exploits the hydrogen protons of the water molecules within the patient and is an excellent modality for the evaluation of soft tissues, ligamentous structures, joint capsule, and the proximal femoral physis. MRI can provide a plethora of information regarding the health and integrity of the

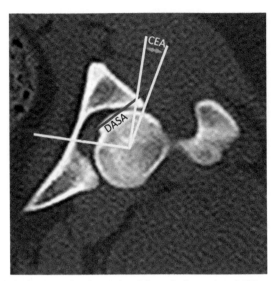

Fig. 11. Various hip indices can be determined from 2-dimensional CT images. Here the CEA and DASA are shown. To determine these values, a line is drawn along the horizontal axis of the pelvis to the center of the femoral head. A second line is drawn from the center of the femoral head to the acetabular rim. The CEA (*green*) is the angle between the acetabular rim and a line perpendicular to pelvic axis. The DASA (*red*) is the angle between the horizontal pelvic axis and the acetabular rim.

subchondral bone with greater sensitivity than other modalities and is currently considered the best noninvasive method for the assessment of articular cartilage.[57] However, factors such as cost, time, required expertise, and need for general anesthesia likely preclude the frequency of the application of this modality with regard to its use in juvenile canine patients for the evaluation of hip dysplasia.

Conventional MRI sequences such as short tau inversion recovery, T1-weighted fast spoiled gradient echo, or T2* imaging are ideal for the evaluation of osseous structures, acetabular cup morphology, femoral head symmetry, and the proximal femoral physes (**Fig. 12**). With proper positioning aids and foam padding, weight-bearing with stress can be simulated within a large body coil with the dog positioned in sternal recumbency. A stifle angle of approximately 135° and the pelvic axis at approximately 100 to 110° to the z-axis of the magnet can aid in this simulation.

Conventional magnetic resonance (MR) sequences do not provide a comprehensive assessment of articular cartilage due to limitations related to spatial resolution and biologic functional information.[57] Two emerging MR methodologies that provide high-resolution evaluation of the cartilage matrices and their physiologic properties include delayed gadolinium-enhanced MRI of cartilage (dGEMRIC) and T2 mapping.[58] When used with gadolinium-based contrast agents in conjunction with T1-weighted spin-echo inversion recovery pulse sequences, dGEMRIC is an advanced and more sensitive protocol acquisition for the assessment of glycosaminoglycan (GAG) density. A loss of charge density within the articular cartilage is often associated with early osteoarthrosis.[58,59] With dGEMRIC imaging, an anionic gadolinium-based contrast agent is given intravenously followed by 15 to 30 minutes of exercise. The MR images are acquired approximately 2 hours later.[60] The agent distributes within the cartilage following active patient movement during the preimaging interim in a quantity that is

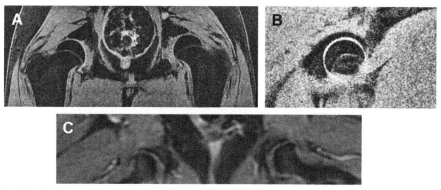

Fig. 12. Unenhanced, T1-weighted fast spoiled gradient echo, transverse (*A*) and sagittal (*B*) images of a normal, juvenile, purpose-bred hound. Although not routinely used for evaluating the canine pelvis for dysplastic changes, this modality can provide anatomic and physiologic information regarding the subchondral bone and periarticular margins. Note the discernible, isointense (to muscle), proximal femoral physis. (*C*) Enhanced, 3D, reconstructable, dorsal, T1-weighted fast spoiled gradient echo image of an 8-year-old, mixed breed dog with moderate, bilateral coxofemoral osteoarthrosis. Note the angular, periarticular osteophytic proliferation along the femoral head. These findings are not uncommonly encountered in patients undergoing MR imaging of the lumbosacral junction or the perineal region.

inversely proportional to the GAG content of the interrogated cartilage. The distribution of contrast is high in degraded cartilage void of GAGs, and conversely, low in healthy cartilage where GAGs are abundant.[58,60] Special software is needed for the generation of T1 color maps that reflect the GAG quantification. In people, color-coded T1 mapping has been shown to be useful for determining cartilage health and can be a positive predictor of surgical outcome following periacetabular osteotomy compared with radiography.[61]

T2-weighted imaging is highly sensitive to water content and tissue hydration.[58] Organized type II collagen fibers are associated with healthy cartilage and water content. Disruption of the cartilaginous matrices and anisotropy of these fibers leads to an increase in water molecule content and interaction, which increase the T2-weighted relaxation times.[57] These T2 relaxation times increase linearly with cartilage damage. Therefore, T2 mapping increases the T2 sensitivity for detecting cartilage damage.[57] The use of both T2 mapping and dGEMRIC studies may enhance future studies of cartilage degeneration associated with canine hip dysplasia and aid in the selection of surgical candidates for juvenile surgical interventions such as the TPO.

ARTHROSCOPY

Although more invasive than diagnostic imaging techniques, arthroscopy can be used to evaluate the coxofemoral joint with the advantage of being able to detect joint and cartilage damage before the onset of radiographic sings of osteoarthritis.[20] Holsworth and colleagues[10] demonstrated that approximately 50% of dogs without radiographic signs of osteoarthritis had moderate to severe cartilage lesions seen arthroscopically. Many surgeons agree that the presence of cartilage damage represents a contraindication for performing corrective osteotomies when treating hip dysplasia (such as with the TPO procedure). Therefore, arthroscopy is often used as a diagnostic tool for improved assessment of the surface of the articular cartilage before surgical interventions. (Please see Francisco Guevara and Samuel P. Franklin's article, "Triple Pelvic Osteotomy and Double Pelvic Osteotomy," in this issue for examples of arthroscopic images of the hip.)

SUMMARY

Diagnostic imaging is a principal method used to diagnose canine hip dysplasia. As evident by the myriad of methods available, no test is perfect, and practitioners must understand the limitations of the modality they are using. Traditional hip-extended radiographs remain the most used method for evaluation and are useful as a screening tool and for detection of radiographic signs of osteoarthritis. However, additional diagnostic methods such as PennHip distraction radiography have been shown to improve sensitivity of laxity detection, allow for more objective means of evaluation, and further aid in prediction of future osteoarthritis development in younger animals. Future studies using more advanced techniques such as CT and MRI may further improve the ability to diagnose and treat hip dysplasia patients, improve the understanding of the disease process, and potentially aid in decreasing the prevalence of the disease through improved selective breeding.

REFERENCES

1. Powers MY, Karbe GT, Gregor TP, et al. Evaluation of the relationship between Orthopedic Foundation for Animals' hip joint scores and PennHIP distraction index values in dogs. J Am Vet Med Assoc 2010;237(5):532–41.
2. Schelle GB. Some new diseases in the dog. Am Kennel Gazette 1935;52:25.
3. Riser WH. Producing diagnostic pelvic radiographs for canine hip dysplasia. J Am Vet Med Assoc 1962;141:600.
4. Owens JM, Biery NA. Radiographic interpretation for the small animal clinician. Baltimore (MD): Williams & Wilkins; 1999.
5. Mayhew PD, McKelvie PJ, Biery DN, et al. Evaluation of a radiographic caudolateral curvilinear osteophyte on the femoral neck and its relationship to degenerative joint disease and distraction index in dogs. J Am Vet Med Assoc 2002;220(4): 472–6.
6. Morgan JP. Canine hip dysplasia: significance of early bony spurring. Vet Radiol Ultrasound 1987;28:2.
7. Powers MY, Biery DN, Lawler DF, et al. Use of the caudolateral curvilinear osteophyte as an early marker for future development of osteoarthritis associated with hip dysplasia in dogs. J Am Vet Med Assoc 2004;225(2):233–7.
8. Risler A, Klauer JM, Keuler NS, et al. Puppy line, metaphyseal sclerosis, and caudolateral curvilinear and circumferential femoral head osteophytes in early detection of canine hip dysplasia. Vet Radiol Ultrasound 2009;50(2):157–66.
9. Szabo SD, Biery DN, Lawler DF, et al. Evaluation of a circumferential femoral head osteophyte as an early indicator of osteoarthritis characteristic of canine hip dysplasia in dogs. J Am Vet Med Assoc 2007;231(6):889–92.
10. Holsworth IG, Schulz KS, Kass PH, et al. Comparison of arthroscopic and radiographic abnormalities in the hip joints of juvenile dogs with hip dysplasia. J Am Vet Med Assoc 2005;227(7):1091–4.
11. Henricson B, Norberg I, Olsson SE. On the etiology and pathogenesis of hip dysplasia: a comparative review. J Small Anim Pract 1966;7:673.
12. Riser WH. The dysplastic hip joint: its radiographic and histologic development. Vet Radiol Ultrasound 1973;14:35–40.

13. Heyman SJ, Smith GK, Cofone MA. Biomechanical study of the effect of coxofemoral positioning on passive hip joint laxity in dogs. Am J Vet Res 1993;54(2): 210–5.

14. Smith GK, Biery DN, Gregor TP. New concepts of coxofemoral joint stability and the development of a clinical stress-radiographic method for quantitating hip joint laxity in the dog. J Am Vet Med Assoc 1990;196(1):59–70.

15. Karbe GT, Vanderhoff K, Runge JJ, et al. Canine hip dysplasia screening: precision and predictive accuracy of the Australian hip scoring method. In: Proceedings of the 36th Annual Conference of the Veterinary Orthopedic Society. Steamboat Springs (CO), February 28–March 6, 2009. p. 24.

16. Paster ER, LaFond E, Biery DN, et al. Estimates of prevalence of hip dysplasia in Golden Retrievers and Rottweilers and the influence of bias on published prevalence figures. J Am Vet Med Assoc 2005;226:387.

17. Verhoeven GEC, Coopman F, Duchateau L, et al. Interobserver agreement on the assessability of standard ventrodorsal hip-extended radiographs and its effect on agreement in the diagnosis of canine hip dysplasia and on routine FCI scoring. Vet Radiol Ultrasound 2009;50:259.

18. Fortrie RR, Verhoeven G, Broeckx B, et al. Intra-and interobserver agreement on radiographic phenotype in the diagnosis of canine hip dysplasia. Vet Surg 2015; 44(4):467–73.

19. Willis MB. A review of the progress in canine hip dysplasia control in Britain. J Am Vet Med Assoc 1997;210:1480.

20. Smith GK, Karge GT, Angello KA, et al. Pathogenesis, diagnosis, and control of canine hip dysplasia. In: Tobais KM, Johnson SA, editors. Veterinary surgery: small animal, vol. 1, 1st edition. St Louis (MO): Saunders/Elsevier; 2012. p. 824–48.

21. Tomlinson JL, Cook JL. Effects of degree of acetabular rotation after triple pelvic osteotomy on the position of the femoral head in relationship to the acetabulum. Vet Surg 2002;31(4):398–403.

22. Skurková L, Hluchý M, Lacková M, et al. Relation of the Norberg angle and position of the femoral head centre to the dorsal acetabular edge in evaluation of canine hip dysplasia. Vet Comp Orthop Traumatol 2010;23(6):433–8.

23. Tomlinson JL, Johnson JC. Quantification of measurement of femoral head coverage and Norberg angle within and among four breeds of dogs. Am J Vet Res 2000;61(12):1492–500.

24. Gold RM, Gregor TP, Huck JL, et al. Effects of osteoarthritis on radiographic measures of laxity and congruence in hip joints of Labrador Retrievers. J Am Vet Med Assoc 2009;234:1549.

25. Popovitch CA, Smith GK, Gregor TP, et al. Comparison of susceptibility for hip dysplasia between Rottweilers and German Shepherd dogs. J Am Vet Med Assoc 1995;206:648.

26. Runge JJ, Kelly SP, Gregor TP, et al. Distraction index as a risk factor for osteoarthritis associated with hip dysplasia in four large dog breeds. J Small Anim Pract 2010;51:264.

27. Smith GK, Gregor TP, Rhodes WH, et al. Coxofemoral joint laxity from distraction radiography and its contemporaneous and prospective correlation with laxity, subjective score, and evidence of degenerative joint disease from conventional hip-extended radiography in dogs. Am J Vet Res 1993;54:1021.

28. Smith GK, Mayhew PD, Kapatkin AS, et al. Evaluation of risk factors for degenerative joint disease associated with hip dysplasia in German Shepherd dogs,

Golden Retrievers, Labrador Retrievers, and Rottweilers. J Am Vet Med Assoc 2001;219:1719.

29. Adams WM, Dueland RT, Meinen J, et al. Early detection of canine hip dysplasia: comparison of two palpation and five radiographic methods. J Am Anim Hosp Assoc 1998;34:339.

30. Smith GK, Hill CM, Gregor TP, et al. Reliability of the hip distraction index in two-month-old German Shepherd dogs. J Am Vet Med Assoc 1998;212:1560.

31. Smith GK, Lawler DF, Biery DN, et al. Comparison of primary osteoarthritis of the hip with the secondary osteoarthritis of canine hip dysplasia. In: Proceedings of the 36th Annual Conference of the Veterinary Orthopedic Society. Steamboat Springs (CO), February 28–March 6, 2009. p. 23.

32. Gatineau M, Dupuis J, Beauregard G, et al. Palpation and dorsal acetabular rim radiographic projection for early detection of canine hip dysplasia: a prospective study. Vet Surg 2012;41(1):42–53.

33. Kealy RD, Lawler DF, Ballam JM, et al. Five-year longitudinal study on limited food consumption and development of osteoarthritis in coxofemoral joints in dogs. J Am Vet Med Assoc 1997;210:222.

34. Smith GK, Paster ER, Powers MY, et al. Lifelong diet restriction and radiographic evidence of osteoarthritis of the hip joint in dogs. J Am Vet Med Assoc 2006;229: 690.

35. Farese JP, Todhunter RJ, Lust G, et al. Dorsolateral subluxation of hip joints in dogs measured in a weight-bearing position with radiography and computed to-mography. Vet Surg 1998;27:393.

36. Smith GK, Popovitch CA, Gregor TP, et al. Evaluation of risk factors for degenerative joint disease associated with hip dysplasia in dogs. J Am Vet Med Assoc 1995;206:642.

37. Flückiger MA, Friedrich GA, Binder H. A radiographic stress technique for evaluation of coxofemoral joint laxity in dogs. Vet Surg 1999;28:1.

38. Slocum B, Devine T. Dorsal acetabular rim radiographic view for evaluation of the canine hip. J Am Anim Hosp Assoc 1990;26:289–96.

39. Prieru WD. Coxarthrosis in the dog: part 1: normal and abnormal biomechanics of the hip joint. Vet Surg 1980;9:145–9.

40. Weigel JP, Wasserman JF. Biomechanics of the normal and abnormal hip joint. Vet Clin North Am Small Anim Pract 1992;22:513–28.

41. DeJardin LM, Perry RL, Arnoczky SP. The effect of triple pelvic osteotomy on the articular contact area of the hip joint in dysplastic dogs: as in vitro experimental study. Vet Surg 1998;27:194–202.

42. Devin-Slocum T, Slocum B. Radiographic characteristics of hip dysplasia. In: Bojrab MJ, editor. Current techniques in small animal surgery. 4th edition. Baltimore (MD): Williams and Wilkins; 1998. p. 1145–51.

43. Trumpatori BJ, Mathews KG, Roe SR, et al. Radiographic anatomy of the canine coxofemoral joint using the dorsal acetabular rim (DAR) view. Vet Radiol Ultrasound 2003;44(5):526–32.

44. Meomartino L, Fatone G, Potena A, et al. Morphometric assessment of the canine hip joint using the dorsal acetabular rim view and the centre-edge angel. J Small Anim Pract 2002;43(1):2–6.

45. Renberg WC, Hoskinson J. A method for visualizing the dorsal acetabular rim and the coverage of the femoral head. Vet Comp Orthop Traumatol 2001;14(3):151–5.

46. Slocum B, Devin-Slocum T. Pelvic osteotomy. In: Bojrab MJ, editor. Current techniques in small animal surgery. 4th edition. Baltimore (MD): Williams and Wilkins; 1998. p. 1159–65.

47. Charette B, Dupuis J. Palpation and dorsal acetabular rim radiographic view for early detection of canine hip dysplasia. Vet Comp Orthop Traumatol 2001;14(3): 125–32.

48. Graf R. The diagnosis of congenital hip-joint dislocation by the ultrasonic compound treatment. Arch Orthop Trauma Surg 1980;97:117.

49. Mahan ST, Katz JN, Kim Y. To screen or not to screen? A decision analysis of the utility of screening for developmental dysplasia of the hip. J Bone Joint Surg Am 2009;91:1705.

50. Adams WM, Dueland RT, Daniels R, et al. Comparison of two palpation, four radiographic and three ultrasound methods for early detection of mild to moderate canine hip dysplasia. Vet Radiol Ultrasound 2000;41:484.

51. Fischer A, Flöck A, Tellhelm B, et al. Static and dynamic ultrasonography for the early diagnosis of canine hip dysplasia. J Small Anim Pract 2010;51:582.

52. Greshake RJ, Ackerman N. Ultrasound evaluation of the coxofemoral joints of the canine neonate. Vet Radiol Ultrasound 1993;34:99.

53. O'Brien RT, Dueland RT, Adams WC, et al. Dynamic ultrasonographic measurement of passive coxofemoral joint laxity in puppies. J Am Anim Hosp Assoc 1997;33:275.

54. Fujiki M, Misumi K, Sakamoto H. Laxity of canine hip joint in two positions with computed tomography. J Vet Med Sci 2004;66:1003.

55. Lopez MJ, Lewis BP, Swaab ME, et al. Relationships among measurements obtained by use of computed tomography and radiography and scores of cartilage microdamage in hip joints with moderate to severe joint laxity of adult dogs. Am J Vet Res 2008;69:362.

56. Andronescu AA, Kelly L, Kearney MT, et al. Associations between early radiographic and computed tomographic measures and canine hip joint osteoarthritis at maturity. Am J Vet Res 2015;76(1):19–27.

57. Gold GE, Chen CA, Koo S, et al. Recent advances in MRI of articular cartilage. AJR Am J Roentgenol 2009;193(3):628.

58. Wucherer KL, Ober CP, Conzemius MG. The use of delayed gadolinium enhanced magnetic resonance imaging of cartilage and T2 mapping to evaluate articular cartilage in the normal canine elbow. Vet Radiol Ultrasound 2012;53(1): 57–63.

59. Dudda M, Young KJ. Delayed gadolinium enhanced MRI of cartilage (dGEMRIC) in HIP Dysplasia. Magentom Flash 2007;1:22–3.

60. Burstein D, Velyvis J, Scott KT, et al. Protocol issues for delayed Gd (DTPA) enhanced MRI (dGEMRIC) for clinical evaluation of articular cartilage. Magn Reson Med 2001;45(1):36–41.

61. Cunningham T, Jessel R, Zurakowski D, et al. Delayed gadolinium-enhanced magnetic resonance imaging of cartilage to predict early failure of Bernese periacetabular osteotomy for hip dysplasia. J Bone Joint Surg Am 2006;88(7): 1540–8.

Canine Hip Dysplasia Screening Within the United States

Pennsylvania Hip Improvement Program and Orthopedic Foundation for Animals Hip/Elbow Database

Jennifer K. Reagan, DVM

KEYWORDS

• PennHIP • OFA • Canine hip dysplasia • Osteoarthritis • Estimated breeding values

KEY POINTS

- High passive hip laxity, as measured by PennHIP distraction index, has been associated with the development of osteoarthritis; however, the hip-extended radiographic view is unreliable for evaluation of passive hip laxity.
- Hip-extended view radiographs are useful for evaluating for the presence of osteoarthritis, which is age dependent but cannot predict future development of osteoarthritis.
- In addition to being a more accurate measure of passive laxity, PennHIP distraction index has a higher heritability than OFA hip scoring and a continuous ratio scale rather than an ordinal grading scale. These attributes may make PennHIP a preferable hip-screening tool for breeding populations.
- Both PennHIP and OFA hip scoring can be used to improve hip phenotypes through breeding, but are more powerful tools when incorporated into estimated breeding values.

INTRODUCTION

Hip dysplasia is the most commonly diagnosed orthopedic condition in the canine.[1] However, canine hip dysplasia (CHD) is mainly a radiographic diagnosis because many dogs that have radiographic changes associated with CHD do not display clinical signs related to the disease. Radiographically, the generally accepted definition of CHD is the presence of hip subluxation and/or hip osteoarthritis (OA).[1] Clinical signs

The author has nothing to disclose.
Department of Veterinary Clinical Medicine, University of Illinois College of Veterinary Medicine, 1008 West Hazelwood Drive, Urbana, IL 61802, USA
E-mail address: jkreaga2@illinois.edu

associated with CHD include pain on hip range of motion, decreases in range of motion of the hip, and lameness.[1] These clinical signs tend to have a bimodal distribution related to age and become most apparent in young dogs (6–12 months) and then again in older dogs.[1] Because clinical signs related to CHD can be severely debilitating and the disease has been shown to have a genetic basis, many radiographic screening programs have been developed in an attempt to decrease the prevalence of the disease within breeding programs.[1]

In the United States, the 2 most commonly implemented canine hip screening programs are the Pennsylvania Hip Improvement Program (PennHIP) and the Orthopedic Foundation for Animals Hip/Elbow Database (OFA). These screening programs have fundamental differences in their method of hip screening as well as criteria for inclusion within the database. The goal of this article is to provide a comprehensive review of the PennHIP and OFA hip screening programs while highlighting their methodological differences and the scientific data supporting the use of these programs in the screening of CHD for breeding programs. As the radiographic techniques of these programs are related to other CHD screening programs worldwide and in the development of estimated breeding values (EBVs), these topics are also briefly discussed.

ORTHOPEDIC FOUNDATION FOR ANIMALS HIP/ELBOW DATABASE METHODOLOGY

The OFA was founded in 1966 with the goal of lowering the incidence of CHD through collation/distribution of information and establishment of control programs and research funding.[2] This goal has since expanded to include many other common orthopedic and nonorthopedic diseases of dogs and cats, such as elbow dysplasia, congenital heart disease, and many others.[2] For CHD, the OFA uses the standard radiographic ventrodorsal hip-extended view (HEV) to evaluate for radiographic

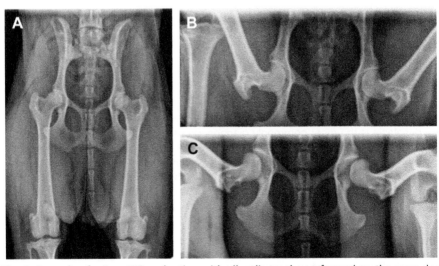

Fig. 1. Example of a PennHIP evaluation with all radiographs performed on the same dog and on the same day. (*A*) HEV performed in the same manner as recommended by OFA. (*B*) Compression view. (*C*) Distraction view. Notice that the subluxation between the HEV and the distraction view is markedly different demonstrating the amount of passive laxity that may not be apparent on the HEV.

changes associated with CHD. Guidelines for positioning of this view include the following (**Fig. 1**A):

- Use of ventrodorsal view with the hind limbs extended and parallel to each other
- Maintain symmetry/proper orientation of the pelvis
- Include the wings of the ilium and stifles/patellas within the radiograph

Specifically, the hips are evaluated for a combination of subluxation, conformational abnormalities, and evidence of OA. The scoring system is listed in **Table 1**. Dogs receiving grades excellent to fair are considered to have "normal" hips, and the variation in grading is based on the presence of "minimal to minor" subluxation/conformation changes.[3] A borderline grade is essentially a nondiagnosis (ie, no consensus on normal or dysplastic). Grades mild to severe are dogs that are considered to have dysplastic hips. To evaluate for evidence of OA and conformation abnormalities consistent with dysplasia, 9 sites of the hip are evaluated[4]:

- Craniolateral acetabular rim
- Cranial acetabular margin
- Femoral head
- Fovea capitis
- Acetabular notch
- Caudal acetabular rim
- Dorsal acetabular margin
- Junction of femoral head and neck
- Trochanteric fossa

Table 1
Orthopedic Foundation for Animals Hip/Elbow Database grading system

Number	OFA Grade	Description[a]
1	Excellent	Superior conformation Almost complete coverage of femoral head
2	Good	Slightly less than superior conformation Good coverage of the femoral head
3	Fair	Minor irregularities of the hip Minor joint incongruency Slightly shallow acetabulum
4	Borderline	No consensus on dysplastic vs normal Greater incongruency than a "fair" hip No OA changes Anatomic variant that cannot be distinguished from OA
5	Mild	Significant subluxation, partial coverage femoral head Shallow acetabulum Usually no arthritic changes
6	Moderate	More significant subluxation, femoral head barely covered OA/remodeling/sclerosis along the femoral neck, head and acetabular rim
7	Severe	Severe subluxation, part or complete loss of coverage of the femoral head Large amounts of OA

All grades are subjectively evaluated in relation to breed, sex and age.
[a] Based on the description provided on the OFA Web site (OFA. An Examination of Hip Grading. 2016. Accessed May 29, 2016).

THE HIP-EXTENDED VIEW AND HIP DYSPLASIA

The HEV is the most commonly used radiographic projection for CHD screening worldwide. The HEV is the radiographic image used in the United States by the OFA; however, other hip scoring systems based on the HEV are used by various organizations, including the Fédération Cynologique Internationale (used in Europe, parts of South America, and Asia) and British Veterinary Association/Kennel Club program (used in the United Kingdom, Australia, and New Zealand).[5] In 1961, a panel convened by the American Veterinary Medical Association established the radiographic positioning and description of the HEV. Since then, this radiograph has been widely used to evaluate for the presence of OA and as such changes consistent with OA have been well described.[1] However, to the author's knowledge, no studies have shown subjective grading of the HEV to be predictive for the development of future OA. Likewise, although the HEV has been shown to be a valuable tool in evaluating for the presence of OA, it can severely underestimate hip laxity (see **Fig. 1**).[1] Maximum lateral displacement of the hip occurs with the limbs in a standing position. Extension and internal rotation of the hips, as occurs with the HEV, can cause spiral tensioning of the fibrous elements of the joint capsule, decreasing the apparent magnitude of laxity.[6] In a study comparing laxity present on the HEV to that of the PennHIP distraction view, the distraction view always showed a greater amount of laxity (mean hip-extended index [HEI] 0.17, mean distraction index [DI] 0.44).[7] The importance of hip laxity lies in one of the prevailing concepts behind the pathogenesis of CHD, which is that hip laxity is the underlying cause of pain and leads to the secondary development of OA.[1] In an effort to quantify laxity on the HEV, measurements such as Norberg angle (NA) have been developed. Although NA can provide an objective measure of subluxation, it remains restricted in its ability to measure subluxation due to the inherent limitations of HEV.

Another major criticism of hip scoring based on the HEV is the variation in interobserver and intraobserver error in the reporting of these scores. The average concordance rate reported by OFA is 74%.[8] The interobserver error improves when the 7-point grading system is reduced to a 3-point grading system (normal, borderline, dysplastic) with the interobserver error being 93.4% to 94.9%[5]; however, this greatly limits distinguishing variations between hip phenotypes. Another study reported a 31% to 68% interobserver error.[5]

PENNSYLVANIA HIP IMPROVEMENT PROGRAM METHODOLOGY

The PennHIP was created in 1993 with the goal of developing a more accurate measurement of subluxation/passive hip laxity and therefore an improved method of canine hip screening founded in evidence-based medicine.[1] In the PennHIP method, 3 radiographic projections are performed: the standard HEV, the compression view, and the distraction view (see **Fig. 1**). The HEV is the same view as performed for OFA evaluation and is used for evaluation of OA development. The compression view is used to evaluate the concentricity of the joint, whereas the distraction view is used to measure passive laxity via the DI.[6] In the distraction view, the femurs are levered against a device (distractor) that causes the femoral head to displace laterally from the acetabulum. The DI is this distance of displacement divided by the radius of the femoral head to normalize the measurement of displacement to the size of the dog. Therefore, the DI is a measure of maximum passive laxity of the joint with a DI of 0 representing absolute joint congruity and a DI of 1 representing complete joint luxation.[6] The proposed advantages of the PennHIP method over the HEV method include the following: accurate measurement of passive laxity, minimization of radiographic positioning artifacts that affect the ability to measure laxity on HEV using NA, and evaluation of hip dysplasia using a ratio scale rather than ordinal or interval scale.[6]

A DI of less than 0.3 is considered to be ideal hip conformation and shows that the hip has minimal laxity/subluxation as well as minimal to no risk of future development of OA.[1] As the DI increases, the amount of laxity increases.[1] Generally, DI of 0.3 to 0.5, 0.5 to 0.7, and greater than 0.7 can be considered to represent mild, moderate, and severe laxity, respectively; however, these intervals have not been strictly defined.[1] DI is breed specific.[9–11] When the DI is reported, the DI for the hip with the greatest laxity is given as well as the percentile that the DI decreases within based on breed.[1] Dogs are only officially called dysplastic if evidence of OA is present on the HEV, whereas the DI addresses the level of subluxation.[1] In OFA hip scoring criteria, hips can be dysplastic based on the level of subluxation without the presence of OA, which is an important difference between PennHIP and OFA scoring. The features of OA evaluated on the PennHIP HEV are similar to those evaluated by OFA and are subjectively graded as mild, moderate, or severe. Generally, PennHIP recommends considering dogs for breeding that have a DI within or greater than the 60th percentile for that breed (ie, the 40% of the population with the least amount of laxity) and that do not have evidence of OA.[12] This recommendation is made to continue to apply selection pressure while avoiding severe restriction of the gene pool because some breeds have few animals that fall within the ideal hip category of less than 0.3.

OTHER SPECIFIC DIFFERENCES BETWEEN ORTHOPEDIC FOUNDATION FOR ANIMALS HIP/ELBOW DATABASE AND PENNSYLVANIA HIP IMPROVEMENT PROGRAM METHODOLOGY
Age of Official Scoring

Dogs must be 2 years of age to receive an official OFA score, whereas dogs between 4 months and 2 years of age will be given a preliminary score. Between 1993 and 2003, the mean age of dogs evaluated for official OFA scores declined from 33 months to 26.5 months.[13] This decline shows that generally OFA scores are performed at a relatively young age, which may impact hip scoring as OA is an age-related process. With preliminary scoring, reliability of the diagnosis of CHD decreases as the scores become closer to fair or mild CHD; therefore, it has been recommended that dogs with these scores have the radiographs repeated at 24 months of age.[14]

Official PennHIP scores are given as early as 4 months of age. Radiographs taken before 16 weeks will be given an unofficial score; however, this score may not be reflective of the true amount of hip laxity present. In a study evaluating German shepherd dogs, it was shown that radiographs performed at 8 weeks of age were not sufficiently reliable to predict DI at 4 and 12 months of age.[15] In this group of dogs, the DIs at 4 months of age were similar to the DIs at 12 months of age.[15] Likewise, a different study showed that DI performed at 6.5 to 9 weeks was not associated with OA development.[16] Because DI is one of the main criteria for consideration for juvenile pubic symphysiodesis, this lack of repeatability is a concern and area for further research because dogs are often tested before 16 weeks of age.

Training Required and Radiographic Evaluation

One of the advantages of OFA scoring is the ease of performing the radiographs. Because no additional training or equipment is required, cost is also usually less. For OFA scoring, the HEV is reviewed by 3 board-certified radiologists, and a consensus is made on the score. If 2 reviewers give a higher score (ie, 2 good and 1 fair), then the higher score is chosen as the final grade. Likewise, if a dog receives an excellent, good, and fair score, the dog will be given the middle grade of good.

Interestingly, based on the OFA Web site, it cannot be determined how a dog given 2 fair grades and 1 good grade would be graded overall.[3] In contrast, the PennHIP method requires the practitioner to undergo additional training as well as prove through a series of test radiographs that they are able to reliably perform the technique. Another difference is that one evaluator rather than the consensus of 3 evaluators determines the PennHIP DI and level of OA.

Database

Self-selection bias is present within the OFA because owners can choose whether to submit radiographs taken by the veterinarian. In a study evaluating submission bias, it was found that 92% of dogs with dysplastic hips were not submitted to the OFA for evaluation; however, 50% of normal dogs were also not submitted, suggesting that this bias occurs in both directions.[11] This self-selection bias may underestimate the proportion of dogs that have CHD. In a study evaluating OFA submissions between 1989 and 2003, a sex bias was noted with male dogs having a small but significant increase in receiving excellent and good grades compared with female dogs.[13] PennHIP has attempted to eliminate this bias by making it mandatory to submit all PennHIP radiographs that are performed for evaluation, which maintains the integrity of the database and allows for less bias within the scientific reports derived from the database. However, potential bias is present in both databases related to breed popularity, push by breeding organizations, and the underlying reason for hip evaluation. Another difference in the databases is that the OFA results are published within the public OFA disease database (dysplastic results are not published without owner permission), whereas the PennHIP database is private.

DISTRACTION INDEX AND CANINE HIP DYSPLASIA

In the process of creating the DI, biomechanical studies were performed to find the optimal positioning of the hips to determine maximal passive laxity.[6,17] It was found that maximal lateral hip displacement occurred with $10°$ of external rotation, $10°$ of extension, and $20°$ of abduction, which is similar to positioning during the stance phase.[17] The repeatability of DI measurements has been evaluated within and between examiners.[18] Overall, the repeatability is very high with the interclass correlation coefficients within examiners being 0.85 to 0.97 and between examiners being 0.75 to 0.95.[18]

DI has been correlated with CHD development in multiple studies.[9,10,19–21] The susceptibility of development of CHD based on DI has been shown to be breed dependent.[9,10,22] For example, in one study, German shepherd dogs were more susceptible to the development of OA at a given DI than Rottweilers with the overall risk of OA development being 6.4 times greater for German shepherd dogs.[22] Similar results were found when comparing these dogs with Golden retrievers and Labrador retrievers with German shepherd dogs having a 4.95 times the risk of OA development compared with the other 3 breeds.[9] Conversely, sight hounds such as Greyhounds and Borzois are known to have a large population with a DI <0.3 and are generally resistant to the development of hip OA. Although the joint laxity estimated with NA on the HEV can decrease with development of OA, DI appears to be relatively unaffected by the onset of OA.[23] However, when the compression index (similar measurement method as DI but performed on the compression view) is evaluated, it increases with onset of OA.[23] The compression view shows acetabular depth, the center of joint rotation, and the overall concentricity of the joint.[6] Therefore, an increase in compression index would be consistent with loss of joint congruity and the ability of the hip to be fully seated within the joint.

STUDIES COMPARING ORTHOPEDIC FOUNDATION FOR ANIMALS HIP/ELBOW DATABASE TYPE HIP SCORING AND PENNSYLVANIA HIP IMPROVEMENT PROGRAM

Only one study has directly compared PennHIP DI results and official OFA hip scores.[24] This study found that 80% (293 of 367 dogs) evaluated as normal by OFA had a DI >0.3, whereas all dysplastic dogs had a DI of greater than 0.3.[24] It concluded that many dogs deemed normal via OFA were susceptible to OA development based on DI, and that this could reduce the ability to eliminate CHD through breeding. The study also reconfirmed that evaluation of laxity on the HEV is poor and underestimates the true amount of passive laxity present based on DI. It is worth noting that there was a significant association between OFA scoring category and mean DI with the mean DI increasing as OFA scores worsened. However, the DI range within each category was wide; therefore, these scores are not equivalent and cannot be substituted.

One prospective longitudinal study comparing DI, OFA type scoring, and NA at 4, 6, 12, 24, and 36 months of age[21] found that DI had the highest agreement in scores over time, whereas the OFA type scoring had the lowest agreement (intraclass correlation coefficient 0.55–0.91 compared with 0.06–0.39, respectively).[21] Another longitudinal study followed 48 Labrador retrievers over their lifetime.[20] Radiographs (HEV) scored using OFA's established criteria were taken at 4, 6, 8, 12, and 18 months of age and then at 2, 3, and 5 years of age, and then yearly until death. PennHIP radiographs were taken at 2 years of age. The major findings of the study were that OFA type hip scoring is a poor predictor of the development of CHD because 55% of dogs graded as normal at 2 years of age developed radiographic evidence of CHD by the end of life, whereas 92% developed histologic evidence.[20] All dogs in the study were considered susceptible to OA development based on DI and 98% of these dogs developed OA based on radiography (67%) or histopathology (96%).[20] For OFA hip scores at 2 years of age, there was only one false positive in this study, whereas there was a high false negative rate (44%).[20] Because false negatives represent animals graded as normal that go on to develop CHD, this would imply this method is poor at predicting CHD later in life and would allow many dogs in the breeding pool with genetics predisposing CHD. The converse has been a common criticism of PennHIP, because some studies have reported a high false positive rate as opposed to the above finding of 2 false positive dogs based on histopathology.[2,20,25,26] These studies however did not follow dogs to the end of life (one ending as early as 12 months), and therefore, the false positive rate reported may be inappropriately high given that OA is age dependent. The lifetime study concluded that the phenotype of the OFA hip score was greatly influenced by environmental factors (diet), whereas DI was not, which suggests DI has higher heritability.[20] The drawback of this study was that all animals were deemed susceptible to CHD and OA development based on DI; therefore, false/true negatives could not be determined.

PennHIP and OFA scores have also been evaluated in relation to the presence of cartilage lesions. In one study, 30-month-old mixed breed hounds were evaluated by various radiographic methods (PennHIP and OFA) and various computed tomographic measurements. Histologic evaluation of the joints was performed immediately after imaging to derive a cartilage score, which represented the cumulative presence of various histologic changes associated with OA. The study found that, of the radiographic methods, the PennHIP OA score (scored as mild, moderate, or severe OA) had the strongest correlation with cartilage score. However, both OFA and PennHIP radiographic methods had a good correlation with cartilage score.[27]

HIP SCREENING AND THE PREDICTIVE VALUE FOR OSTEOARTHRITIS DEVELOPMENT

OA is an age-dependent condition and represents one of the greatest challenges in CHD screening. DI has been shown to be a risk factor for development of OA in several studies.[22,28] Initial correlations of DI to the development of CHD showed that dogs with a DI <0.4 had a high probability for normal hips, whereas development of CHD was highly probable with a DI >0.7.[19] In 48 Labrador retrievers, the odds of OA development were 2.2 times higher for every 0.1 increase in DI.[20] Likewise, dogs with a DI <0.4 did not develop OA until 12 years of age.[20] Interestingly, in dogs evaluated longitudinally over their lifetime for CHD, all dogs diagnosed with subluxation were diagnosed by 2 years of age, whereas all new cases of CHD after 2 years of age were due to OA development.[20] This finding lends further credence to the concept that hip laxity is an inherent characteristic of CHD, whereas OA development appears secondary and can be influenced by environmental factors such as diet. It also highlights the dilemma of using the HEV early in life as a predictor for later development of CHD because OA development is age and environment dependent.

CANINE HIP DYSPLASIA IMPROVEMENT OVER GENERATIONS: HIP-EXTENDED VIEW AND ORTHOPEDIC FOUNDATION FOR ANIMALS HIP/ELBOW DATABASE

Studies evaluating for improvement in hip phenotype using the HEV as a breeding guideline have had mixed results with some studies[5,29] claiming no substantial improvement, whereas others state the opposite.[8,13,30] The general consensus seems to be that at best only modest improvement has occurred. Specifically using the OFA database, there are several studies that have attempted to evaluate for evidence of improvement in the canine hip phenotype.[30] A study comparing the percentage of hips graded as excellent in dogs whelped between 1972 and 1980 and 1989 and 1992 found an increase from 7.8% to 10.6%.[13] When evaluating dogs from 1989 to 2003, there was a significant increase in proportion of dogs graded as good and excellent from 1993 compared with 2003 and an increase in odds of receiving an excellent grade compared with the 1989 to 1992 cohort.[30] However, the exact odds ratios were not given but appeared to be relatively low based on a graph within the paper, oscillating between 0.9 and 1.6 and between 1993 and 2003.

Hou and colleagues[8] in 2010 looked at genetic improvement in Labrador retrievers evaluated by the OFA between 1970 and 2007 that were between 24 and 60 months of age. They showed that the hip scores improved from an average of 2.02 to 1.9 over 30 years with 2 being equal to good and 1 being equal to excellent. Although they concluded that genetic improvement had occurred, they recommended basing breeding on EBVs (see later discussion) as the heritability score of the HEV phenotype used by OFA appeared low (0.21). It was also stated that DI would likely lead to faster improvement as DI has a higher heritability.

ESTIMATED BREEDING VALUE

CHD is a polygenetic disease, and no single phenotype has been shown to completely correlate with the genotype.[30] Selective breeding using PennHIP or OFA is limited in utility because it does not account for other factors that make an animal a valuable breeding candidate, nor does it account for the hip scores of relatives. EBV for a phenotypic trait (such as OFA or PennHIP scores) can be calculated using mixed model equations. Because EBV incorporates information related to pedigree and genetically related traits, they can more accurately estimate the genetic merit of an individual compared with its contemporaries.[29,31] Therefore, knowing the EBV for desired traits allows for improved selection of breeding animals and potentially faster genetic improvement.

Heritability and selection pressure are related because phenotypes with higher heritability will cause faster change when the same selection pressure is placed. Generally, a heritability of 1 means that 100% of the phenotypic appearance can be explained by genetic variation. A heritability of 0.5 means that 50% of the phenotype can be related to genetic variation, whereas 50% is related to other factors such as environment. A heritability of greater than 0.15 to 0.2 has been reported to produce enough selection pressure to effect change.[32] Based on the OFA records, the estimated heritability of OFA scoring for the Labrador retriever is 0.21.[8] Estimated heritability for OFA type scoring of other breeds has been shown to range from 0.22 to 0.76.[29,33–36] The heritability of DI has been shown to be generally higher at 0.61 to 0.83,[36,37] which could improve the rate of CHD phenotypic change. In addition to increased heritability, EBVs are improved with knowledge of the pedigree, results for a given hip score/desired trait, and the number of dogs evaluated, which highlights the need for a database to track these results as well as EBV.

An article documenting the breeding program for Seeing Eye Inc showed that significant improvement in hips occurred over 5 generations using subjective hip scoring, similar to that used with OFA, along with EBV. However, after 4 generations, the scores began to cluster, reducing a 9-point grading scale to a 3-point grading scale. The author stated that they planned to use DI as a means to further differentiate dogs within the breeding program.[38] To date, no studies have been published documenting the effect of the use of EBV incorporating DI on a population of dogs.

It is important to remember that breeding based on PennHIP DI or OFA scoring selects for a phenotype (ie, that specific radiographic appearance). This phenotype is not necessarily related to other traits of the disease such as risk for clinical signs. Currently, there are no published studies that have directly correlated either of these radiographic phenotypes with clinical signs of hip dysplasia. Based on a study that evaluated genetic correlations for DI, NA, OFA type scoring, and dorsolateral subluxation (DLS), it was found that OFA type scoring and NA were highly correlated and DI and DLS were highly correlated.[36] However, measurements of laxity (DI and DLS) and measures based off of the HEV only exhibited moderate genetic correlation, which suggests possible different genetic influences.[36]

SUMMARY

CHD is a complex, polygenic disease that is associated with hip subluxation and development of OA. Screening programs have been established with the goal of hip improvement; however, minimal progress has been documented. The underlying reasons are likely multifactorial and include the hip screening method used, whether EBVs were used, access to/knowledge about breeding stock, and the relative concern about CHD related to other desired traits. When evaluating the single HEV used by OFA versus the 3 radiographic views and associated DI used by PennHIP for CHD screening, the scientific evidence greatly supports the use of the DI and PennHIP method.

REFERENCES

1. Tobias KM, Johnston SA. Veterinary surgery: small animal. St Louis (MO): Elsevier; 2012.
2. Keller GG, Dziuk E, Bell JS. How the orthopedic foundation for animals (OFA) is tackling inherited disorders in the USA: using hip and elbow dysplasia as examples. Vet J 2011;189(2):197–202.

3. OFA. An Examination of Hip Grading. 2016. Available at: http://www.ofa.org/hd_grades.html. Accessed May 29, 2016.

4. OFA. The OFA's Hip Radiograph Procedures. 2016. Available at: http://www.offa.org/hd_procedures.html. Accessed May 29, 2016.

5. Verhoeven G, Fortrie R, Van Ryssen B, et al. Worldwide screening for canine hip dysplasia: where are we now? Vet Surg 2012;41(1):10–9.

6. Smith GK, Biery DN, Gregor TP. New concepts of coxofemoral joint stability and the development of a clinical stress-radiographic method for quantitating hip joint laxity in the dog. J Am Vet Med Assoc 1990;196(1):59–70.

7. Kapatkin AS, Gregor TP, Hearon K, et al. Comparison of two radiographic techniques for evaluation of hip joint laxity in 10 breeds of dogs. J Am Vet Med Assoc 2004;224(4):542–6.

8. Hou Y, Wang Y, Lust G, et al. Retrospective analysis for genetic improvement of hip joints of cohort Labrador retrievers in the United States: 1970-2007. PLoS One 2010;5(2):e9410.

9. Smith GK, Mayhew PD, Kapatkin AS, et al. Evaluation of risk factors for degenerative joint disease associated with hip dysplasia in German Shepherd Dogs, Golden Retrievers, Labrador Retrievers, and Rottweilers. J Am Vet Med Assoc 2001;219(12):1719–24.

10. Runge JJ, Kelly SP, Gregor TP, et al. Distraction index as a risk factor for osteoarthritis associated with hip dysplasia in four large dog breeds. J Small Anim Pract 2010;51(5):264–9.

11. Paster ER, LaFond E, Biery DN, et al. Estimates of prevalence of hip dysplasia in Golden Retrievers and Rottweilers and the influence of bias on published prevalence figures. J Am Vet Med Assoc 2005;226(3):387–92.

12. PennHIP AIS. Selection Pressure in Breeding. 2016. Available at: http://info.antechimagingservices.com/pennhip/navigation/owner-breeder-information/selective-breeding.html. Accessed May 29, 2016.

13. Kaneene JB, Mostosky UV, Padgett GA. Retrospective cohort study of changes in hip joint phenotype of dogs in the United States. J Am Vet Med Assoc 1997;211(12):1542–4.

14. Corley EA, Keller GG, Lattimer JC, et al. Reliability of early radiographic evaluations for canine hip dysplasia obtained from the standard ventrodorsal radiographic projection. J Am Vet Med Assoc 1997;211(9):1142–6.

15. Smith GK, Hill CM, Gregor TP, et al. Reliability of the hip distraction index in two-month-old German shepherd dogs. J Am Vet Med Assoc 1998;212(10):1560–3.

16. Adams WM, Dueland RT, Daniels R, et al. Comparison of two palpation, four radiographic and three ultrasound methods for early detection of mild to moderate canine hip dysplasia. Vet Radiol Ultrasound 2000;41(6):484–90.

17. Heyman SJ, Smith GK, Cofone MA. Biomechanical study of the effect of coxofemoral positioning on passive hip joint laxity in dogs. Am J Vet Res 1993;54(2):210–5.

18. Smith GK, LaFond E, Gregor TP, et al. Within- and between-examiner repeatability of distraction indices of the hip joints in dogs. Am J Vet Res 1997;58(10):1076–7.

19. Lust G, Williams AJ, Burton-Wurster N, et al. Joint laxity and its association with hip dysplasia in Labrador retrievers. Am J Vet Res 1993;54(12):1990–9.

20. Smith GK, Lawler DF, Biery DN, et al. Chronology of hip dysplasia development in a cohort of 48 Labrador retrievers followed for life. Vet Surg 2012;41(1):20–33.

21. Smith GK, Gregor TP, Rhodes WH, et al. Coxofemoral joint laxity from distraction radiography and its contemporaneous and prospective correlation with laxity,

subjective score, and evidence of degenerative joint disease from conventional hip-extended radiography in dogs. Am J Vet Res 1993;54(7):1021–42.

22. Popovitch CA, Smith GK, Gregor TP, et al. Comparison of susceptibility for hip dysplasia between Rottweilers and German shepherd dogs. J Am Vet Med Assoc 1995;206(5):648–50.

23. Gold RM, Gregor TP, Huck JL, et al. Effects of osteoarthritis on radiographic measures of laxity and congruence in hip joints of Labrador Retrievers. J Am Vet Med Assoc 2009;234(12):1549–54.

24. Karbe GT, Biery DN, Gregor TP, et al. Radiographic hip joint phenotype of the Pembroke Welsh Corgi. Vet Surg 2012;41(1):34–41.

25. Harasen G. Assessing the dysplastic hip. Can Vet J 2009;50(4):427–8.

26. Ohlerth S, Busato A, Rauch M, et al. Comparison of three distraction methods and conventional radiography for early diagnosis of canine hip dysplasia. J Small Anim Pract 2003;44(12):524–9.

27. Lopez MJ, Lewis BP, Swaab ME, et al. Relationships among measurements obtained by use of computed tomography and radiography and scores of cartilage microdamage in hip joints with moderate to severe joint laxity of adult dogs. Am J Vet Res 2008;69(3):362–70.

28. Smith GK, Popovitch CA, Gregor TP, et al. Evaluation of risk factors for degenerative joint disease associated with hip dysplasia in dogs. J Am Vet Med Assoc 1995;206(5):642–7.

29. Soo M, Worth A. Canine hip dysplasia: phenotypic scoring and the role of estimated breeding value analysis. N Z Vet J 2015;63(2):69–78.

30. Kaneene JB, Mostosky UV, Miller R. Update of a retrospective cohort study of changes in hip joint phenotype of dogs evaluated by the OFA in the United States, 1989-2003. Vet Surg 2009;38(3):398–405.

31. Wilson BJ, Nicholas FW, James JW, et al. Estimated breeding values for canine hip dysplasia radiographic traits in a cohort of Australian German Shepherd dogs. PLoS One 2013;8(10):e77470.

32. Wilson B, Nicholas FW, Thomson PC. Selection against canine hip dysplasia: success or failure? Vet J 2011;189(2):160–8.

33. Leighton EA, Linn JM, Willham RL, et al. A genetic study of canine hip dysplasia. Am J Vet Res 1977;38(2):241–4.

34. Hedhammar A, Olsson SE, Andersson SA, et al. Canine hip dysplasia: study of heritability in 401 litters of German Shepherd dogs. J Am Vet Med Assoc 1979; 174(9):1012–6.

35. Reed AL, Keller GG, Vogt DW, et al. Effect of dam and sire qualitative hip conformation scores on progeny hip conformation. J Am Vet Med Assoc 2000;217(5): 675–80.

36. Zhang Z, Zhu L, Sandler J, et al. Estimation of heritabilities, genetic correlations, and breeding values of four traits that collectively define hip dysplasia in dogs. Am J Vet Res 2009;70(4):483–92.

37. Ginja MM, Silvestre AM, Ferreira AJ, et al. Passive hip laxity in Estrela Mountain Dog–distraction index, heritability and breeding values. Acta Vet Hung 2008; 56(3):303–12.

38. Leighton EA. Genetics of canine hip dysplasia. J Am Vet Med Assoc 1997; 210(10):1474–9.

Conservative Management of Hip Dysplasia

Tisha A.M. Harper, DVM, MS, CCRP

KEYWORDS

- Osteoarthritis • Nonsteroidal anti-inflammatory drugs • Physical therapy
- Weight management • Conservative management

KEY POINTS

- When developing a conservative management protocol for dogs with hip dysplasia (HD), a multimodal approach, which is tailored to the individual pet, should be used.
- Conservative management plans should be re-evaluated periodically and adjusted as needed, because a patient's needs change with time.
- Immature dogs with HD presenting with acute lameness at 3 months to 6 months of age can have spontaneous improvement in hind limb function once they reach maturity.
- Conservative management of HD often primarily involves treatment of osteoarthritis (OA). Nonsteroidal anti-inflammatory drugs (NSAIDs) are the mainstay of treatment of hip OA.
- There are many nonpharmacologic treatment options available for the conservative management of HD. Client education is an important component of the management protocol.

INTRODUCTION

HD is a common orthopedic condition seen in dogs characterized by laxity of the coxofemoral joint.[1] This can lead to significant pain and lameness due to subluxation, stretching of the joint capsule, and microfractures of the acetabulum in immature patients and OA in the mature patients.[1–3] Both conservative and surgical options are available to treat immature as well as mature patients with clinical signs attributed to HD.[1,2] Immature patients typically display hind limb lameness acutely between 3 months and 6 months of age. Spontaneous improvement in hind limb function, however, occurs in a large number of immature dogs with HD once they reach maturity.[2,4,5] In a study comparing long-term results of conservative treatment to 2 surgical procedures (triple pelvic osteotomy and femoral head and neck excision), the investigators did not find a marked difference in ground reaction forces between

Disclosure Statement: The author has nothing to disclose.
Department of Veterinary Clinical Medicine, University of Illinois College of Veterinary Medicine, 1008 West Hazelwood Drive, Urbana, IL 61802, USA
E-mail address: taharper@illinois.edu

dogs in the conservative treatment group and those in the triple pelvic osteotomy and control groups.[5] Barr and colleagues[4] also evaluated the long-term results of conservative management of 68 immature dogs in which HD was diagnosed at an early age. They found that 76% had minimal gait abnormalities at a mean of 4.5 years later. This spontaneous improvement may have been due to healing of microfractures of the dorsal acetabular rim as well as improved joint congruity and stability secondary to remodeling of the articular components and thickening of the joint capsule.[6] It is, therefore, reasonable to initially manage immature patients conservatively and determine their response to conservative management. Mature patients tend to have a history of progressive hind limb lameness due to progressive OA and can also be managed conservatively.[3] Conservative treatment is almost always the first step in management of patients with clinical signs attributed to HD. If they fail to respond, surgery should be considered. HD has a multifactorial mode of inheritance; therefore, even though a pet may be genetically predisposed to the disease, the severity and development of clinical signs can be altered by changing environment and lifestyle.[2,7] In the immature dog, conservative management involves exercise restriction, weight control, analgesics, and physical therapy.[8] In mature dogs, conservative management is focused on treating OA. The general goals of conservative treatment are to alleviate pain and discomfort, maintain function and range of motion (ROM) of the hip, and regain normal activity, thereby restoring quality of life. Another goal is to slow the progression of the disease, if possible, without causing significant side effects that ultimately affect quality of life.[3,9] To achieve these goals, conservative management focuses on weight and body condition score, pain control, strengthening periarticular muscles, limiting excessive joint stress, maintaining or improving joint ROM and proprioception, maintaining or improving cartilage health, and limiting inflammation.[9] Treatment can be divided into different phases depending on the age at presentation (ie, alleviating either acute or chronic clinical signs).[3] Treatment in the acute phase involves strict rest, anti-inflammatory medications, and additional analgesics as needed. Introduction to physical therapy modalities, in particular those that alleviate pain and inflammation, can also be instituted.[1] Long-term management includes dietary, activity, and lifestyle changes to maintain quality of life and function.

PATIENT EVALUATION OVERVIEW

Management protocols for HD should be designed for the individual patient. Therefore, a comprehensive clinical evaluation, including gait assessment, neurologic evaluation, and evaluation for other orthopedic disease, is necessary prior to making treatment recommendations. NSAIDs are commonly used to manage the pain and inflammation associated with HD; therefore, comprehensive health panels are needed to screen pets prior to implementing NSAID treatment. Radiographs are important for assessing the severity of hip laxity/incongruity and the severity of secondary OA; however, decisions on treatment should be based predominantly on history, clinical signs on presentation, and the results of physical examination because there is poor correlation between radiographic findings, joint lesions, and clinical function in dogs with HD.[4,10,11] Factors to consider when developing a treatment plan include age at initial diagnosis, level of discomfort, physical examination findings, radiographic findings, breed and temperament, client expectations for the pet, and owner finances.[3,12] Conservative treatment can be divided into short-term treatment and long-term treatments.[1] Short-term treatment is aimed at the acutely affected patient to quickly address pain and decrease inflammation.[3]

PHARMACOLOGIC TREATMENT OPTIONS
Nonsteroidal Anti-inflammatory Drugs and Other Analgesics

NSAIDs are the mainstay of treatment to alleviate the pain and inflammation associated with HD.[13,14] In OA there is degradation of the articular cartilage with a resulting loss of proteoglycans from the extracellular matrix and the subsequent release of inflammatory mediators and degradative enzymes.[13,15] The disease is not confined to the cartilage because synovial inflammation and capsular fibrosis, changes in the metabolism and architecture of subchondral bone, and periarticular osteophyte and enthesophyte formation also occur. Proinflammatory cytokines (eg, interleukin 1 and tumor necrosis factor α) play a role in the inflammatory process.[13] Cell membrane damage results in the production of arachidonic acid by the action of phospholipase A2 on cell membrane phospholipids. Metabolism of arachidonic acid by cyclooxygenase (COX) enzymes results in the release of different eicosanoids, including prostaglandin E_2 (PGE_2), thromboxane A_2, prostacyclin, and lipoxins.[14] There are 2 well-known forms of COX, COX-1 and COX-2. A variant of COX-1 (COX-3) has also been identified in the dog; however, its activity is still uncertain.[14,16,17] NSAIDs inhibit 1 or more steps in the metabolism of arachidonic acid by inhibiting COX enzymes, thus inhibiting the production of prostaglandins and thromboxane and their associated effects.[13] PGE_2 is important in vasodilation, sensitization of nociceptors, and protection of the gastrointestinal (GI) tract by increased mucus production, vasodilation, and thus increased blood flow to the gastric mucosa, reduced gastric acid secretion, increased secretion of bicarbonate in the duodenum, and increased turnover of mucosal cells.[14,17] Thromboxane A2 plays a role in promoting coagulation and blood clot formation whereas prostacyclin inhibits platelet aggregation.[14] The action of lipoxygenases (LOXs) on arachidonic acid results in the formation of leukotrienes, which also promotes the inflammatory response.[13] Inhibition of COX enzymes by NSAIDs may result in a shift in arachidonic acid metabolism to the LOX pathway, resulting in increased production of leukotrienes. This might explain why most NSAIDs available for use in small animal patients may not provide complete relief of pain and inflammation.[13,18] One of the relatively newer NSAIDs, tepoxalin, inhibits both COX-1 and COX-2 as well as 5-LOX activity; however, it is not currently available in the United States. A study by Lascelles and colleagues[19] looked at the expression of COX-1, COX-2, and 5-LOX in joint tissue from dogs with naturally occurring hip OA and found increased expression of COX-2 in joints with OA compared with tissues from healthy joints. 5-LOX was also increased and they concluded that COX-2 and 5-LOX seem appropriate treatment targets for palliating clinical signs of OA. COX enzymes are also thought to play a role in central sensitization and the pain experienced in OA; NSAIDs may also act by preventing central sensitization.[13] There are several NSAIDs currently licensed for chronic use in dogs that are commonly used for short-term and long-term treatments of OA. They include carprofen, deracoxib, etodolac, firocoxib, mavacoxib, ketoprofen, meloxicam, phenylbutazone, robenacoxib, tepoxalin, and tolfenamic acid. Preference should be given to COX-1–sparing drugs because they seem to have less adverse GI effects than COX-1 selective compounds, for example, aspirin.[14,17] Dosage forms, approved indications, and dosages can be found elsewhere in the literature.[1,13,14,20] A multimodal pharmacologic approach to treating OA is important, particularly during the initial treatment phase, during acute flareups, and to facilitate physical therapy. NSAIDs are often combined with other analgesics to diminish pain and maximize comfort. There is a synergistic effect when NSAIDs and opioids are combined, such that the dose of opioid may be reduced when treating mild to moderate pain.[18] Analgesics that can be considered and used in conjunction with NSAIDs include amantadine, gabapentin, tricyclic antidepressants (eg, amitriptyline and clomipramine), tramadol, acetaminophen, and codeine.[13,20] These are briefly discussed.

Tramadol is a centrally acting synthetic opioid analgesic that is often used to treat mild to moderate pain.[21] It has multiple effects: it inhibits the reuptake of norepinephrine and serotonin, has an effect on α_2-adrenergic receptors in pain pathways, and has mild opiate effects through μ-opioid receptor action.[20] The main metabolites evaluated in dogs are O-desmethyltramadol (M1), N-desmethyltramadol (M2) and N,O-didesmethyltramadol (M5).[22] The M1 metabolite is thought to be responsible for its opiate effects; however, the concentration has been shown to be low in some studies and is thought to play only a minor role in the analgesic effect of tramadol, suggesting that its nonopioid activity is primarily responsible for analgesia.[20,21,23,24] Tramadol is well tolerated in dogs and dose-related sedation is the main side-effect. Seizures can occur at higher doses.[20,22] Tramadol should not be administered with other drugs that affect the reuptake or metabolism of serotonin.[25]

Gabapentin is a γ-aminobutyric acid (GABA) analog that is used in small animal patients both as an analgesic and an anticonvulsant. It is used to treat chronic neuropathic pain. The mechanism of action is thought to be blockage of the N-type voltage-dependent calcium channels on neurons. It does not bind to GABA receptors. Gabapentin also increases the brain concentrations of GABA although the mechanism by which this occurs is not clearly understood.[20,25] Gabapentin has been used in conjunction with NSAIDs to treat chronic OA pain; however, studies assessing its efficacy as an analgesic in small animal patients are lacking. Sedation and ataxia are the main side effects and are seen when used at higher dosages.[20,25]

Acetaminophen is an effective analgesic agent. Its mechanism of action is not completely understood. Acetaminophen has been categorized as a COX-3 inhibitor; however, newer research suggests that its activity is mediated by the activation of serotonin receptors due to the interplay of transient receptor potential vanilloid type 1 receptors.[16,26] Combinations of acetaminophen with an opiate, for example, codeine, may be more effective for treating moderate pain in dogs,[20] although this effect has not been proved and further studies are warranted.[26] Acetaminophen is toxic in cats because they are unable to secrete its metabolites.[20]

Codeine is a μ-opioid agonist analgesic. The active metabolite codeine-6-glucuronide is thought to provide an analgesic effect in dogs; however, the efficacy of codeine as a sole analgesic agent in small animals is uncertain.[20,25]

Amantadine (N-methyl-D-aspartate [NMDA] receptor antagonist) has been used as an adjunct analgesic for treating chronic OA in dogs.[27] It is an antiviral drug with analgesic effect thought to be mediated by its NMDA antagonist activity, which results in antagonizing central pain sensitization and decreases tolerance to opioids. Amantadine should not be used as a sole analgesic agent but may work well in combination with other pain medications, for example, NSAIDs, opioids, and gabapentin.[25] One clinical study assessing the effectiveness of amantadine combined with meloxicam demonstrated a beneficial effect[27]; however, further evaluation of appropriate dosages based on a recent pharmacologic study has been suggested.[28]

Clinical trials evaluating tricyclic antidepressants for the treatment of pain in dogs are lacking. Their analgesic effect is due to multiple mechanisms: NMDA antagonism, serotonin and norepinephrine receptor uptake inhibition, voltage-gated sodium channel blockade, enhanced activity of adenosine, and GABA$_B$ receptors and anti-inflammatory effects.[25]

Weight Loss Pharmaceuticals

Diet and exercise are important for weight loss; however, in some patients, particularly very obese patients, results take a long time and require a long-term commitment by the owner, which can often be frustrating. These pets are often unable to exercise initially due to excess body weight and the pain of OA. Weight loss pharmaceuticals may be considered a health management tool in managing obesity in patients with OA.[29] Mitratapide and dirlotapide are microsomal triglyceride transfer protein inhibitors, which, when administered orally in dogs, decrease the uptake of dietary lipids.[29] Mitratapide has been shown to result in weight loss by primarily targeting adipose tissue.[29] Dirlotapide also decreases food intake in a dose-dependent manner, which is thought to be its primary mechanism for weight loss.[30] An additional advantage of weight-loss pharmaceuticals is that they can be used in the short-term in conjunction with the existing diet in a well-designed weight-reduction program.[30]

Corticosteroids

Corticosteroids reduce the inflammation associated with OA by inhibiting the activity of phospholipase A2.[15,31] Although this provides immediate relief of pain due to the decrease in inflammation, there is still uncertainty about its effects on articular cartilage.[32] A systematic review of the literature revealed methodological weaknesses in many animal studies evaluating the effects of corticosteroids on articular cartilage, making it difficult to draw definitive conclusions.[32] Corticosteroids can be administered orally or locally by intra-articular injection and both routes of administration have been shown to be effective in reducing early OA changes in experimentally induced OA in dogs, without having adverse effects on normal articular cartilage.[13,15,33,34] The protective effect was more pronounced for intra-articular triamcinolone hexacetonide administration compared with oral prednisone in 1 study.[33] In vitro, corticosteroids have been shown to have a dose-dependent effect on proteoglycan synthesis in normal articular cartilage in horses and dogs.[35] Beneficial effects of corticosteroids have also been demonstrated, with the proposed mechanism inhibition of cartilage matrix metalloproteinases and inflammatory cytokines.[35] Intra-articular corticosteroids have also been combined with local anesthetics to treat the clinical effects of OA.[36] There are many safer options for the treatment of OA in dogs and the general recommendation is that corticosteroids should be reserved for patients with end-stage disease that are refractory to all other treatments and for whom surgical intervention is not an option. Corticosteroids should not be administered concurrently with NSAIDs because the risk of severe GI adverse effects is increased. Adverse effects on the kidney and platelet function have also been reported with this combination of drugs.[14,18] When used to treat OA, low doses of corticosteroids should be administered locally by intra-articular injection of long-acting preparations, such as triamcinolone and methylprednisolone.[13,33,35,36] Triamcinolone has been shown experimentally to have the least deleterious effects on the cartilage and synovium.[36] Currently most veterinarians follow the recommendations for humans, that is, 1 injection every 6 weeks and no more than 3 to 4 intra-articular injections in a year.[13] Prior to administrationn, steps must be taken to ensure that joint infection is not present. After administration, patients should be restricted from heavy joint loading and exercise for several weeks to protect any remaining cartilage.[37] Potential complications associated with intraarticular injections in general are cartilage damage and joint sepsis. Oral corticosteroids can be used short term to treat acute flare ups in pets unresponsive to other therapy. Long-term use should be avoided due to systemic side effects for example, polyuria, polyphagia, polydipsia, GI ulceration, and muscle atrophy.[15,31]

Nutraceuticals and Other Disease-modifying Agents

- Polysulfated glycosaminoglycans (PSGAG) may be beneficial in treating OA.[38] The exact mode of action is not clear; however, PSGAG is thought to inhibit proteolytic enzymes, decrease the production of inflammatory mediators, and accelerate extracellular matrix production by stimulation of chondrocytes and synoviocytes.[38] An in vitro study evaluating the effect of PSGAG on DNA content and proteoglycan metabolism in normal and osteoarthritic canine articular cartilage explants found that PSGAG inhibited proteoglycan degradation in osteoarthritic explants and maintained or increased DNA content. The investigators noted that if the results of the study extended to in vivo use, PSGAG treatment may modify the progression of OA by maintaining chondrocyte viability or stimulating chondrocyte division by protecting against extracellular matrix degradation.[39] PSGAG is typically administered as twice-weekly intramuscular injections for 4 weeks.[20]
- Pentosan polysulfate is a semisynthetic polysulfated xylan isolated from beechwood hemicellulose. Its proposed benefit in the treatment of OA is in promoting the synthesis of cartilage extracellular matrix components and attenuation of cartilage degradation.[40] It also promotes the synthesis of high-molecular-weight hyaluronan by synovial cells. Pentosan polysulfate also has anticoagulant properties and may improve blood flow through the synovium and subchondral bone due to its thrombolytic and lipolytic effects.[40,41] A systematic review by Aragon and colleagues[42] showed a moderate level of comfort for the use of pentosan polysulfate for the treatment of OA in dogs. Further clinical studies are needed to evaluate its efficacy; however, it is associated with a low incidence of side effects.[43] It is administered by subcutaneous injection once a week.
- Hyaluronan is a normal component of synovial fluid and articular cartilage. In arthritic joints the concentrations of hyaluronan decrease, resulting in a decrease in the viscosity of the synovial fluid.[1] Intra-articular injection of hyaluronic acid has been described to treat dogs with hip OA; however, there was no evidence supporting the efficacy of hyaluronan for the treatment of OA in the dog in 2 systematic reviews.[42,44] Newer studies that would not have been included in these systematic reviews suggest a clinical benefit after intra-articular hyaluronic acid injection.[45,46] Further meta-analyses are needed to determine its benefits.
- Glucosamine and chondroitin sulfate – glucosamine is a precursor of the disaccharide unit of glycosaminoglycan. Chondroitin sulfate is a polymer of repeating disaccharide units (galactosamine sulfate and glucuronic acid). They are both components of articular cartilage and have demonstrated bioavailability after oral administration.[47] The veterinary literature is lacking on the effectiveness of either glucosamine or chondroitin sulfate used alone for the treatment of OA; however, they are often combined and administered as dietary supplements. Significant improvements in pain scores and weight bearing have been reported after administration of an oral glucosamine/chondroitin formulation, but no objective evaluation of outcome was done in this study.[47] The investigators also noted that the onset of action was slow, greater than 70 days. These can be administered as supplements or provided in functional foods as part of a complete diet.[13]

- Omega-3 fatty acids (FAs) have been shown to decrease the clinical signs of OA in dogs and can also be provided as a supplement or in a functional food.[13,32,48,49] Supplementation with omega-3 FAs results in an increase in their concentrations in tissues and cell membranes and a corresponding decrease in omega-6 FA concentrations and decreased arachidonic acid production.[48] Omega-3 FAs are also thought to alter the production of eicosanoids to less inflammatory forms and to reduce the expression of cartilage-degrading enzymes, COX-2, and the inducible inflammatory cytokines interleukin 1a and tumor necrosis factor.[32] In a systematic review of the efficacy of nutraceuticals in alleviating the clinical signs of OA, diets supplemented with omega-3 FAs demonstrated a positive effect in ameliorating some of the clinical signs.[32] Supplementation with omega-3 FAs is reportedly associated with few adverse effects.[48,49]

Other disease-modifying agents that have been used to treat OA in dogs include green-lipped mussel, elk velvet antler, and P54FP (turmeric extract).[50–54] There was a moderate level of comfort in 2 systematic reviews in the efficacy of these agents for treating OA in dogs.[42,44]

NONPHARMACOLOGIC TREATMENT OPTIONS

Weight management is an important component in treating dogs with hip OA.[7,13,55,56] In OA, the degrading cartilage does not resist biomechanical stress as effectively as healthy cartilage. As a result, excessive body weight causes additional mechanical stress on joints, hastening the degenerative process. Restricting caloric intake minimizes the prevalence and severity of OA in the coxofemoral joint.[1,7,56] Overweight adult dogs with clinical signs of hip OA fed calorie-restricted diets have been shown to improve significantly after weight loss, at least in the short term.[55,57] Impellizeri and colleagues[55] investigated the effect of a restricted-calorie diet in adult dogs between 6 years and 13 years of age with radiographic evidence and clinical signs of bilateral hip OA. These dogs were at least 10% greater than their ideal bodyweight ranging in weight between 17 kg and 52.7 kg. No additional drug therapy or food supplements were administered for the duration of the study. Significant improvements in clinical signs with weight reduction alone (loss of at least 10% of bodyweight) were noted in the short term, that is, during the period of weight loss (10–19 weeks).[55] Another study investigating the effect of limited food consumption on the incidence of HD in growing dogs found that the dogs that were fed a restricted diet (25% less food compared with the control group fed ad libitum) from 8 weeks to 2 years of age had less radiographic hip joint laxity at any time point compared with litter mates fed ad libitum.[58] When these dogs were evaluated again at 8 years of age, the limit-fed dogs had a significantly lower prevalence and later onset of hip OA compared with controls.[7] Limited food intake is, therefore, an environmental factor that can have a profound effect on the prevalence of OA in the coxofemoral joint in dogs.[7] Weight reduction in overweight pets can be achieved through calorie reduction, eliminating treats and encouraging exercise but may also necessitate the use of prescription diets and weight loss pharmaceuticals. The ultimate goal is to maintain these animals at a lean bodyweight. The target body condition score for dogs is 4.5 (1–9 scale) or 2.5 (1–5 scale).[1] Owners should be instructed to feed for the targeted body weight and that all food, including treats, should be included when calculating daily caloric intake.[1] There is also growing evidence that body fat has metabolic activity that promotes inflammatory reactions within the body, which may contribute to the pathophysiology of OA.[59] Therefore, weight reduction should also have a direct anti-inflammatory effect through the reduction in proinflammatory adipokines.[59]

Exercise restriction is important in the treatment of OA in dogs. Excessive stress on the unhealthy joint cartilage should be limited; however, consistent moderate activity is important for joint health. Regular, controlled, low-impact activities, for example, leash walking, walking in water, and swimming, are beneficial activities for these patients.[9] Controlled exercise should be gradually introduced, particularly in patients that are sedentary or extremely painful. Activity is restricted for 2 weeks to 3 weeks in acutely affected patients to quell the acute inflammation.[3] Pets should be confined to a small space at all times except when taken on limited leash walks outdoors. This can be combined with NSAIDs to decrease the inflammation during the resting period.[3] Active pets may benefit from exercise restriction if exercise is exacerbating the clinical signs of HD, for example, an agility dog may benefit from decreased training or retiring.[60]

Rehabilitation and Physical Therapy

Physical rehabilitation for patients with OA can be challenging because these pets are often very painful, have decreased ROM in the hips, muscle atrophy, and as a result, restricted activity.[61] This is a continuous cycle of progressive loss of muscle mass and strength, which leads to further stress on the painful osteoarthritic joints, leading to further decreases in activity and disability. The goal of physical therapy is to avoid worsening the clinical signs. Therefore, during the early phases of therapy, pharmaceutical therapy is often used to decrease pain and inflammation. Non–weight-bearing types of activities are also often prioritized during early phases of treatment. Other options for managing pain include laser therapy, shockwave therapy, transcutaneous electrical nerve stimulation, heat and cold therapy, therapeutic ultrasound, and massage for muscle spasms.[9,61] **Table 1** is a physical rehabilitation protocol that can be used for conservative management of dogs with HD. (Please see David L. Dycus and colleagues' article, "Physical Rehabilitation for the Management of Canine Hip Dysplasia," in this issue, for a detailed discussion on physical therapy.)

Environmental Modification

Environmental modification is often overlooked as part of the comprehensive treatment protocol for pets with OA. Pets with OA, in particular those with chronic OA, often lose proprioceptive function, making it difficult for them to navigate across slippery surfaces. These pets need to have throw rugs or nonslip mats in the home environment to make it easier for them to get around. Pets with arthritic joints also benefit from supportive orthopedic bedding and ramps to facilitate movement into and out of vehicles or on and off furniture. Keeping them in warm environments and keeping their joints warm on cold days (eg, sweaters) also help with their mobility. These pets also benefit from activities on nonconcussive surfaces, such as grass or sod, instead of more rigid surfaces like concrete. Eliminating or at least minimizing the use of stairs is also helpful.

Regenerative Medicine

The application of regenerative medicine techniques to treat OA in dogs is a rapidly developing field. Mesenchymal stem cells (MSCs) have been most commonly studied and seem to reduce the inflammation associated with OA by decreasing the production of inflammatory cytokines and cartilage-degrading enzymes.[62] MSCs are multipotent adult stem cells that can differentiate into a variety of tissues, including bone, adipose tissue, and cartilage. In dogs, MSCs have been harvested from bone marrow, adipose tissue, muscle, periosteum, and synovium.[62] The anti-inflammatory effects of MSCs injected directly into the joint seem to be short term because the injected

Table 1
Rehabilitation protocol for osteoarthritis of the hip joint

All Treatments Every 6 h	Lameness Score 5/5	Lameness Score 4/5	Lameness Score 3/5	Lameness Score 2/5	Lameness Score 1/5	Lameness Score 0/5
Heat therapy	10 min	10 min	10 min	10 min	10 min	10 min
Massage	5 min	5 min	5 min	5 min	5 min	5 min
Passive ROM (repetitions)[a]	15	15	15	15	15	15
Electrical stimulation[b]	10 min	10 min	10 min	10 min	—	—
Therapeutic exercise: total time	5 min	10 min	15 min	15 min	20 min	20 min
Walk/land treadmill[c]	5 min	10 min	15 min	20 min	20 min	20 min
Balancing	+	+	+	+	+	—
Obstacles	+	+	+	+	+	+
Weaving	+	+	+	+	+	+
Circles	—	—	—	+	+	+
Hills	—	—	—	—	+	+
Stairs	—	—	—	—	—	+
Jog/run	—	—	—	—	—	+
Underwater treadmill	5 min	10 min	15 min	20 min	20 min	20 min
Swimming	—	—	—	—	5–10 min	5–10 min
Cryotherapy	15 min	15 min	15 min	15 min	15 min	15 min

+, Perform modality.
[a] Passive ROM to all joints of the affected limb.
[b] Electrical stimulation to be performed on the semimembranosus/semitendinosus muscle groups in patients with muscle atrophy.
[c] Alternate land treadmill and underwater treadmill during session; do not do both in 1 session. Do land treadmill/walk when at home and institute underwater treadmill 2 to 3 times a week.
From Fossum TW. Small animal surgery. 4th Edition. St Louis (MO): Elsevier Mosby; 2012; with permission.

suspensions of MSCs do not engraft onto cartilage defects. Ongoing studies evaluating the use of scaffolds and matrices for delivery of MSCs into the osteoarthritic joint to support regeneration of damaged tissue show promise. The use of platelet-rich plasma has also shown promise in the treatment of OA in dogs. Platelets are a natural reservoir of growth factors that are thought to directly promote healing and also promote tissue repair through recruitment of stem cells to the site of application.[63–65] Further studies are needed to determine the ideal composition of platelet-rich plasma and its effectiveness in dogs.

COMBINATION THERAPIES

All of the treatment options described in this section are used to either a greater or lesser extent depending on the individual patient as part of a multimodal approach to conservative management. The combination of a weight reduction program and physical therapy, however, for the treatment of lameness in overweight dogs with gait abnormalities attributable to OA has been specifically evaluated.[57] Improvement in clinical signs and weight loss were noted in all dogs. In addition, those dogs receiving intensive physical therapy combined with the calorie restriction had a better outcome/improvement in clinical signs compared with those that only received at-home physical therapy done by the owner.[57]

SURGICAL TREATMENT OPTIONS

There are many surgical treatment options for HD, all of which modify the anatomy of the coxofemoral joint in some way. Some of the surgical procedures for the treatment of HD are discussed in this issue. The surgical procedure recommended depends on the age of the dog and clinical signs. Options for skeletally immature dogs to either prevent the development of clinical signs of HD or prevent or decrease the clinical effects of secondary OA when it occurs include juvenile pubic symphysiodesis and pelvic osteotomies.[66] In mature patients, surgical options are aimed at eliminating OA in the hip and, therefore, are considered salvage procedures. Total hip arthroplasty and femoral head and neck excision are surgical options for mature patients or for immature patients in which other surgical procedures are not an option.[66] The only described surgical procedure that specifically only addresses the pain associated with HD is the coxofemoral denervation procedure.[67] The proposed mechanism of pain relief is by destroying the nerves innervating the joint capsule by curettage of the dorsal acetabular rim.[67] Reports on the effectiveness of the procedure are variable and difficult to compare due to different criteria used for evaluation of dogs postoperatively.[67,68]

COMPLICATIONS

Although NSAIDs can rapidly palliate the symptoms of OA, they can be associated with adverse effects. The most common adverse effects seen with NSAIDs are related to the GI system and may present clinically as vomiting, diarrhea and anorexia.[14,42] GI erosion, ulceration, or perforation may also occur secondary to NSAID usage. Apart from inhibition of prostaglandins, NSAIDs can cause direct irritation to the GI mucosa because many are weak acids. Different NSAIDs should never be administered concurrently because this increases the risk for GI adverse effects.[14] Renal and hepatic toxicity are also reported adverse effects associated with the use of NSAIDs; therefore, screening health panels assessing hepatic and renal function are recommended prior to administration of NSAIDs, particularly in geriatric patients. Health panels should also be re-evaluated periodically during the course of treatment.[14] Caution must also be used when administering NSAIDs to patients with diminished hepatic function because this can decrease the rate of elimination of these drugs and potentially increase GI and renal adverse effects.[14] Individual patients may respond differently to 1 NSAID compared with another; therefore, lack of response to 1 NSAID should prompt the clinician to try an alternative product.[14]

EVALUATION OF OUTCOME AND LONG-TERM RECOMMENDATIONS

Conservative management strategies are aimed at alleviating pain and discomfort, improving ROM, and building muscle mass. Progression of OA, however, still occurs and the severity or rate of progression varies from patient to patient. Pet owners should, therefore, be made aware that other treatment options, such as surgery, may need to be considered if a pet does not respond favorably to conservative management and develops debilitating OA. A review of the literature on the efficacy and safety of long-term use of NSAIDs to treat chronic OA in dogs suggests a clinical benefit with low risk of adverse side effects.[42,69] Reduction in bodyweight is one of the most important components of conservative management of HD. It is often difficult for owners to assess progress on calorie-restricted diets or weight reduction programs; therefore, repeated bodyweight evaluations and follow-up with veterinarians are needed long term to provide encouragement and to ensure that pet owners are on the right track.

SUMMARY/DISCUSSION

Conservative management of HD should use a multimodal approach that is individualized for each patient. The therapy chosen varies depending on factors, such as the age of the patient or stage of the disease. Early institution of medical management, especially weight management, can play an important role in slowing the progression of the disease and improving outcomes. Client education about the disease and the effect/role that environmental factors can play in progression of the disease is critical to management of their pets.

REFERENCES

1. Fossum TW. Small animal surgery. 4th edition. St Louis (MO): Elsevier Mosby; 2012. p. 1305–16.
2. Smith GK, Karbe GT, Agnello KA, et al. Pathogenesis, diagnosis, and control of canine hip dysplasia. In: Tobias KM, Johnston SA, editors. Veterinary surgery small animal. St Louis (MO): Elsevier Saunders; 2012. p. 824–48.
3. Dassler CL. Canine hip dysplasia: diagnosis and nonsurgical treatment. In: Slatter D, editor. Textbook of small animal surgery. 3rd edition. Philadelphia: W B Saunders; 2002. p. 2019–29.
4. Barr ARS, Denny HR, Gibbs C. Clinical hip dysplasia in growing dogs: the long-term results of conservative management. J Small Anim Pract 1987;(28):243–52.
5. Plante J, Dupuis J, Beauregard G, et al. Long-term results of conservative treatment, excision arthroplasty and triple pelvic osteotomy for the treatment of hip dysplasia in the immature dog. Part 2: analysis of ground reaction forces. Vet Comp Orthop Traumatol 1997;(10):130–5.
6. Riser WH. The dysplastic hip joint: its radiographic and histologic development. J Am Vet Radiol Soc 1973;(14):35–50.
7. Kealy RD, Lawler DF, Ballam JM, et al. Evaluation of the effect of limited food consumption on radiographic evidence of osteoarthritis in dogs. J Am Vet Med Assoc 2000;217(11):1678–80.
8. Anderson A. Treatment of hip dysplasia. J small Anim Pract 2011;52(4):182–9.
9. Davidson JR, Kerwin S. Common orthopedic conditions and their physical rehabilitation. In: Millis D, Levine D, editors. Canine rehabilitation and physical therapy. 2nd edition. Elsevier Saunders; 2014. p. 543–78.
10. Read RA. Conservative management of juvenile canine hip dysplasia. Aust Vet J 2000;78(12):818–9.
11. Plante J, Dupuis J, Beauregard G, et al. Long-term results of conservative treatment, excision arthroplasty adn triple pelvic osteotomy for the treatment of hip dysplasia in the immature dog: part 1 radiographic and physical results. Vet Comp Orthop Traumatol 1997;(10):101–10.
12. Rawson EA, Aronsohn MG, Burk RL. Simultaneous bilateral femoral head and neck ostectomy for the treatment of canine hip dysplasia. J Am Anim Hosp Assoc 2005;41(3):166–70.

13. Innes JF. Arthritis. In: Tobias KM, Johnston SA, editors. Veterinary surgery small animal. St Louis (MO): Elsevier Saunders; 2012. p. 1078–111.

14. KuKanich B, Bidgood T, Knesl O. Clinical pharmacology of nonsteroidal anti-inflammatory drugs in dogs. Vet Anaesth Analg 2012;39(1):69–90.

15. Johnston SA, Budsberg SC. Nonsteroidal anti-inflammatory drugs and corticosteroids for the management of canine osteoarthritis. Vet Clin North Am Small Anim Pract 1997;27(4):841–62.

16. Botting RM. Vane's discovery of the mechanism of action of aspirin changed our understanding of its clinical pharmacology. Pharmacol Rep 2010;62(3):518–25.

17. Clark TP. The clinical pharmacology of cyclooxygenase-2-selective and dual inhibitors. Vet Clin North America Small Anim Pract 2006;36(5):1061–85, vii.

18. Mathews KA. Non-steroidal anti-inflammatory analgesics. In: Ettinger SJ, Feldman EC, editors. Textbook of veterinary internal medicine. 7th edition. St Louis (MO): Saunders Elsevier; 2010. p. 608–15.

19. Lascelles BD, King S, Roe S, et al. Expression and activity of COX-1 and 2 and 5-LOX in joint tissues from dogs with naturally occurring coxofemoral joint osteoarthritis. J Orthop Res 2009;27(9):1204–8.

20. Papich MG. Saunders handbook of veterinary drugs: small and large animal. 3rd edition. St Louis (MO): Elsevier Saunders; 2011.

21. KuKanich B, Papich MG. Pharmacokinetics of tramadol and the metabolite O-desmethyltramadol in dogs. J Vet Pharmacol Ther 2004;27(4):239–46.

22. Kukanich B, Papich MG. Pharmacokinetics and antinociceptive effects of oral tramadol hydrochloride administration in greyhounds. Am J Vet Res 2011;72(2):256–62.

23. Benitez ME, Roush JK, KuKanich B, et al. Pharmacokinetics of hydrocodone and tramadol administered for control of postoperative pain in dogs following tibial plateau leveling osteotomy. Am J Vet Res 2015;76(9):763–70.

24. Malek S, Sample SJ, Schwartz Z, et al. Effect of analgesic therapy on clinical outcome measures in a randomized controlled trial using client-owned dogs with hip osteoarthritis. BMC Vet Res 2012;8:185.

25. KuKanich B. Outpatient oral analgesics in dogs and cats beyond nonsteroidal antiinflammatory drugs: an evidence-based approach. Vet Clin North America Small Anim Pract 2013;43(5):1109–25.

26. KuKanich B. Pharmacokinetics and pharmacodynamics of oral acetaminophen in combination with codeine in healthy Greyhound dogs. J Vet Pharmacol Ther 2016;39(5):514–7.

27. Lascelles BD, Gaynor JS, Smith ES, et al. Amantadine in a multimodal analgesic regimen for alleviation of refractory osteoarthritis pain in dogs. J Vet Intern Med 2008;22(1):53–9.

28. Norkus C, Rankin D, Warner M, et al. Pharmacokinetics of oral amantadine in greyhound dogs. J Vet Pharmacol Ther 2015;38(3):305–8.

29. Dobenecker B, De Bock M, Engelen M, et al. Effect of mitratapide on body composition, body measurements and glucose tolerance in obese beagles. Vet Res Commun 2009;33(8):839–47.

30. Wren JA, Gossellin J, Sunderland SJ. Dirlotapide: a review of its properties and role in the management of obesity in dogs. J Vet Pharmacol Ther 2007; 30(Suppl 1):11–6.

31. Cohn LA. Glucocorticoid therapy. In: Ettinger SJ, Feldman EC, editors. Textbook of veterinary internal medicine. 7th edition. St Louis (MO): Saunders Elsevier; 2010. p. 602–8.

32. Vandeweerd JM, Coisnon C, Clegg P, et al. Systematic review of efficacy of nutraceuticals to alleviate clinical signs of osteoarthritis. J Vet Intern Med 2012; 26(3):448–56.

33. Pelletier JP, Martel-Pelletier J. Protective effects of corticosteroids on cartilage lesions and osteophyte formation in the Pond-Nuki dog model of osteoarthritis. Arthritis Rheum 1989;32(2):181–93.

34. Pelletier JP, Martel-Pelletier J. In vivo protective effects of prophylactic treatment with tiaprofenic acid or intraarticular corticosteroids on osteoarthritic lesions in the experimental dog model. J Rheumatol Suppl 1991;27:127–30.

35. Murphy DJ, Todhunter RJ, Fubini SL, et al. The effects of methylprednisolone on normal and monocyte-conditioned medium-treated articular cartilage from dogs and horses. Vet Surg 2000;29(6):546–57.

36. Sherman SL, Khazai RS, James CH, et al. In vitro toxicity of local anesthetics and corticosteroids on chondrocyte and synoviocyte viability and metabolism. Cartilage 2015;6(4):233–40.

37. Farquhar T, Todhunter RJ, Fubini SL, et al. Effect of methylprednisolone and mechanical loading on canine articular cartilage in explant culture. Osteoarthritis Cartilage 1996;4(1):55–62.

38. Fujiki M, Shineha J, Yamanokuchi K, et al. Effects of treatment with polysulfated glycosaminoglycan on serum cartilage oligomeric matrix protein and C-reactive protein concentrations, serum matrix metalloproteinase-2 and -9 activities, and lameness in dogs with osteoarthritis. Am J Vet Res 2007;68(8):827–33.

39. Sevalla K, Todhunter RJ, Vernier-Singer M, et al. Effect of polysulfated glycosaminoglycan on DNA content and proteoglycan metabolism in normal and osteoarthritic canine articular cartilage explants. Vet Surg 2000;29(5):407–14.

40. Henrotin Y, Sanchez C, Balligand M. Pharmaceutical and nutraceutical management of canine osteoarthritis: present and future perspectives. Vet J 2005;170(1): 113–23.

41. Read RA, Cullis-Hill D, Jones MP. Systemic use of pentosan polysulphate in the treatment of osteoarthritis. J small Anim Pract 1996;37(3):108–14.

42. Aragon CL, Hofmeister EH, Budsberg SC. Systematic review of clinical trials of treatments for osteoarthritis in dogs. J Am Vet Med Assoc 2007;230(4):514–21.

43. Hannon RL, Smith JG, Cullis-Hill D, et al. Safety of cartrophen vet in the dog: review of adverse reaction reports in the UK. J small Anim Pract 2003;44(5):202–8.

44. Sanderson RO, Beata C, Flipo RM, et al. Systematic review of the management of canine osteoarthritis. Vet Rec 2009;164(14):418–24.

45. Carapeba GO, Cavaleti P, Nicacio GM, et al. Intra-Articular hyaluronic acid compared to traditional conservative treatment in dogs with osteoarthritis associated with hip dysplasia. Evid Based Complement Alternat Med 2016;2016: 2076921.

46. Nganvongpanit K, Boonsri B, Sripratak T, et al. Effects of one-time and two-time intra-articular injection of hyaluronic acid sodium salt after joint surgery in dogs. J Vet Sci 2013;14(2):215–22.

47. McCarthy G, O'Donovan J, Jones B, et al. Randomised double-blind, positive-controlled trial to assess the efficacy of glucosamine/chondroitin sulfate for the treatment of dogs with osteoarthritis. Vet J 2007;174(1):54–61.

48. Roush JK, Cross AR, Renberg WC, et al. Evaluation of the effects of dietary supplementation with fish oil omega-3 fatty acids on weight bearing in dogs with osteoarthritis. J Am Vet Med Assoc 2010;236(1):67–73.

49. Fritsch D, Allen TA, Dodd CE, et al. Dose-titration effects of fish oil in osteoarthritic dogs. J Vet Intern Med 2010;24(5):1020–6.

50. Rialland P, Bichot S, Lussier B, et al. Effect of a diet enriched with green-lipped mussel on pain behavior and functioning in dogs with clinical osteoarthritis. Can J Vet Res 2013;77(1):66–74.

51. Pollard B, Guilford WG, Ankenbauer-Perkins KL, et al. Clinical efficacy and tolerance of an extract of green-lipped mussel (Perna canaliculus) in dogs presumptively diagnosed with degenerative joint disease. N Z Vet J 2006;54(3):114–8.

52. Bui LM, Bierer TL. Influence of green lipped mussels (Perna canaliculus) in alleviating signs of arthritis in dogs. Vet Ther 2003;4(4):397–407.

53. Moreau M, Dupuis J, Bonneau NH, et al. Clinical evaluation of a powder of quality elk velvet antler for the treatment of osteoarthrosis in dogs. Can Vet J 2004;45(2): 133–9.

54. Innes JF, Fuller CJ, Grover ER, et al. Randomised, double-blind, placebo-controlled parallel group study of P54FP for the treatment of dogs with osteoarthritis. Vet Rec 2003;152(15):457–60.

55. Impellizeri JA, Tetrick MA, Muir P. Effect of weight reduction on clinical signs of lameness in dogs with hip osteoarthritis. J Am Vet Med Assoc 2000;216(7): 1089–91.

56. Kealy RD, Lawler DF, Ballam JM, et al. Five-year longitudinal study on limited food consumption and development of osteoarthritis in coxofemoral joints of dogs. J Am Vet Med Assoc 1997;210(2):222–5.

57. Mlacnik E, Bockstahler BA, Muller M, et al. Effects of caloric restriction and a moderate or intense physiotherapy program for treatment of lameness in overweight dogs with osteoarthritis. J Am Vet Med Assoc 2006;229(11):1756–60.

58. Kealy RD, Olsson SE, Monti KL, et al. Effects of limited food consumption on the incidence of hip dysplasia in growing dogs. J Am Vet Med Assoc 1992;201(6): 857–63.

59. Hamper B. Current topics in canine and feline obesity. Vet Clin North America Small Anim Pract 2016;46(5):785–95.

60. Piermattei DL, Flo GL, DeCamp CE. Handbook of small animal orthopedics and fracture repair. 4th edition. St Louis (MO): Saunders Elsevier; 2006.

61. Henderson AL, Latimer C, Millis D. Rehabilitation and physical therapy for selected orthopedic conditions in veterinary patients. Vet Clin Small Anim 2015; 45:91–121.

62. Whitworth DJ, Banks TA. Stem cell therapies for treating osteoarthritis: prescient or premature? Vet J 2014;202(3):416–24.

63. Corti L. Nonpharmaceutical approaches to pain management. Top Companion Anim Med 2014;29(1):24–8.

64. Franklin SP, Cook JL. Prospective trial of autologous conditioned plasma versus hyaluronan plus corticosteroid for elbow osteoarthritis in dogs. Can Vet J 2013; 54(9):881–4.

65. Fahie MA, Ortolano GA, Guercio V, et al. A randomized controlled trial of the efficacy of autologous platelet therapy for the treatment of osteoarthritis in dogs. J Am Vet Med Assoc 2013;243(9):1291–7.

66. Roush JK. Surgical therapy of canine hip dysplasia. In: Tobias KM, Johnston SA, editors. Veterinary surgery small animal. St Louis (MO): Elsevier Saunders; 2012. p. 849–64.

67. Kinzel S, VonScheven C, Buecker A, et al. Clinical evaluation of denervation of the canine hip joint capsule: a retrospective study of 117 dogs. Vet Comp Orthop Traumatol 2002;15(1):51–6.

68. Lister SA, Roush JK, Renberg WC, et al. Ground reaction force analysis of unilateral coxofemoral denervation for the treatment of canine hip dysplasia. Vet Comp Orthop Traumatol 2009;22(2):137–41.
69. Innes JF, Clayton J, Lascelles BD. Review of the safety and efficacy of long-term NSAID use in the treatment of canine osteoarthritis. Vet Rec 2010;166(8):226–30.

Physical Rehabilitation for the Management of Canine Hip Dysplasia

David L. Dycus, DVM, MS, CCRP[a],*,
David Levine, PT, PhD, DPT, CCRP, Cert DN[b],
Denis J. Marcellin-Little, DEDV[c]

KEYWORDS

- Hip dysplasia • Osteoarthritis • Hip laxity • Therapeutic modalities
- Triple pelvic osteotomy • Juvenile pubic symphysiodesis
- Femoral head and neck ostectomy • Total hip replacement

KEY POINTS

- The goals of rehabilitation at various stages of canine hip dysplasia vary; initially, clinical signs and discomfort are thought to be due to underlying laxity.
- Laxity results in lateralization of the femoral head during the swing phase of the gait with a "catastrophic reduction" of the femoral head into the acetabulum during foot strike.
- Conservative management is centered around maintaining pain control and comfort while improving hip range of motion in extension and muscle mass.
- Surgical therapy focuses on improving femoral head coverage and reducing the development of osteoarthritis or removing the source of discomfort.
- Each aspect of rehabilitation such as manual, therapeutic, and physical modalities follows a multimodal patient-centered approach.

INTRODUCTION

Canine hip dysplasia (CHD) causes diffuse joint inflammation and subsequent coxofemoral osteoarthritis (OA).[1,2] Hip dysplasia was identified in more than 40% of golden retrievers and Rottweilers in 1 report.[3] Hip dysplasia was originally described more than 80 years ago, but its exact etiology remains unknown; however, it is

Disclosure: The authors have nothing to disclose.
[a] Department of Orthopedic Surgery, Veterinary Orthopedic and Sports Medicine Group (VOSM), 10975 Guilford Road, Annapolis Junction, MD 20701, USA; [b] Department of Physical Therapy, University of Tennessee at Chattanooga, 615 McCallie Avenue, Chattanooga, TN 37403, USA; [c] Department of Clinical Sciences, College of Veterinary Medicine, North Carolina State University, NCSU CVM VHC #2563, 1052 William Moore Drive, Raleigh, NC 27607, USA
* Corresponding author.
E-mail address: dldycus@gmail.com

considered multifactorial with both genetic and environmental cues playing a role in its phenotypic expression.[3] The central theme surrounding CHD is hip laxity, which is thought to play a major role in the development of OA. Hip laxity permits subluxation during growth, which results in abnormal development of the acetabulum and femoral head. The repetitive subluxation and reduction lead to excessive cartilage wear and damage to the dorsal acetabular rim, leading to OA. OA progresses over time.[4] Management of CHD is centered around both conservative and surgical therapies, as well as the age of the onset of clinical signs.[4–6] Physical rehabilitation will play a role in the management of CHD, with either conservative or surgical therapies by providing pain relief through strengthening, maintaining range of motion (ROM), promoting optimal weight, and environmental modifications if needed. The purpose of this article is to present the rehabilitation steps that can be implemented to manage CHD at its various stages.

PHYSICAL REHABILITATION IN THE CONSERVATIVE MANAGEMENT OF HIP DYSPLASIA

Although CHD has been analyzed in several hundred scientific publications, few publications discuss the conservative management of OA in dogs, and fewer have assessed the long-term clinical signs and progression of OA.[7] The approach should be multimodal, with goals to improve function, reduce clinical signs of pain, improve hip ROM and strength, and thus potentially slow down or minimize the progression of OA. Given that the goal of conservative management of CHD is aimed at trying to improve the coxofemoral joint environment, many of the recommendations for management are similar to the management of OA. Loss of motion in OA patients results from the development of osteophytes and enthesophytes, thickening of the synovium, and from potential changes in muscle fiber elasticity. Motion should be assessed at regular intervals using goniometry as an objective assessment.[8] Loss of limb strength, core strength, and cardiovascular fitness results from a decrease in spontaneous activity, a decrease in owner-supervised exercise, and a reflex inhibition of muscle contractions (secondary to joint pain).[9] Although OA in dogs is most often diagnosed on radiographs, osteophyte size and severity of clinical signs correlate poorly. As a consequence, the management of OA should not be based on radiographic appearance, but rather on the specific physical limitations of the patient. The goals of conservative management of CHD and the associated OA are accomplished by weight reduction, minimizing joint pain, pharmaceuticals, disease-modifying osteoarthritic agents, manual therapy, therapeutic exercises, and physical modalities. Weight reduction, minimizing joint pain, pharmaceutical, and disease-modifying osteoarthritic agents are covered elsewhere in this issue.

Manual Therapy to Minimize Joint Pain

Nonpharmacologic, antiinflammatory options for peripheral pain management include cold therapy (icing) and massage. Icing provides direct pain relief by decreasing nerve conduction velocity. It also provides secondary pain relief by decreasing edema (itself a source of pain) and decreasing the overactivity of catabolic enzymes in osteoarthritic cartilage.[10,11] Icing should be considered in osteoarthritic patients with flare-ups, after a period of exercise, and before bedtime. Ice cubes or frozen vegetables are not recommended because they have large air pockets that decrease cold conduction. Ice bags filled with ice chips or crushed ice or cold packs provide more effective cold delivery. Most cold packs reach therapeutic temperatures after 2 hours in a freezer. For longhaired patients, place and hold an ice bag or cold pack directly on the pet's arthritic joint or joints and secure it with a self-adhesive band. A towel may be used between the cold pack or bag and the skin in patients with short or no hair. Some cold packs have built-in self-adhesive bands. A neoprene sleeve may also be used to secure a cold pack or bag. Icing should last for 10 to 15 minutes to achieve effective cooling (**Fig. 1**).[10] Most dogs tolerate the treatment, but should not be left unattended. The person applying the ice should make sure the patient is not uncomfortable and that the skin surface feels cold to the touch after icing.

Additional nonpharmacologic options for central pain management include low-level heating, massage, and possibly acupuncture, acupressure, and electroacupuncture. The short-term and long-term effects of massage in companion animals are not known. Massage may decrease myofascial pain and muscle tension.[12] These methods primarily stimulate Aβ sensory fibers with rapid conduction velocities (30–70 m/s), sparing pain fibers with slower conduction velocities: Aδ (12–30 m/s) and C fibers (0.5–3 m/s). Heat is widely considered to positively impact painful OA patients (**Fig. 2**).[11] The use of heat is 2-fold. Low-level heat (elevation of tissue temperature by 1–2°C) relieves pain through the stimulation of nonnociceptive Aβ sensory fibers, as well as the vasodilation and normalization of blood flow. This low-level tissue relaxation may be achieved by keeping osteoarthritic patients in relatively dry and warm temperatures throughout the day (eg, sleeping in heated indoor environments or providing heated beds). More intense heat (elevation of tissue temperature by 3–4°C) is used to increase the effectiveness of stretching while minimizing tissue damage. Intense heating is most often applied by a health care professional using a hot pack that is heated by a hydrocollator or microwave oven. Four layers of dry towels are generally placed between a hot pack and the skin, and heat is generally applied for 10 to 20 minutes.[13] Caution must be used when placing a hot pack on a dog because burns can occur. Initially, the packs may not seem to be excessively hot to the touch, but they can induce thermal damage after several minutes of contact. Furthermore, it is not recommended to use heating pads in place of a hot pack. Checking for excessive redness, skin swelling, or blistering every few minutes during intense heat therapy is important.

Therapeutic Exercises to Minimize Joint Pain, Maintain or Increase Joint Motion

To help with minimizing joint pain and increasing joint motion in the hip, active and passive ROM along with stretching exercises are important (**Fig. 3**). Little is known about the impact of OA on joint motion: dysplastic hips seemingly lose extension but not flexion, dysplastic elbows primarily lose flexion, and arthritic stifles lose

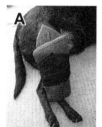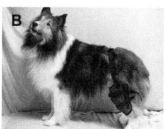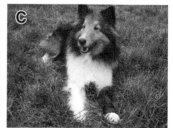

Fig. 1. Limb cryotherapy can be done using (*A*) a cold pack wrapped around the hind limb, (*B*) cryotherapy to the stifle, or (*C*) cryotherapy to the carpus. (*From* Millis D, Levine D. Canine rehabilitation and physical therapy. 2nd edition. Philadelphia: Saunders; 2016. p. 318; with permission.)

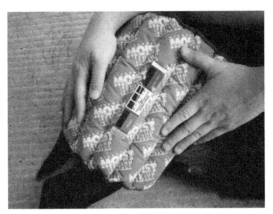

Fig. 2. A hot pack is applied over a dog's hip region. (*From* Millis D, Levine D. Canine rehabilitation and physical therapy. 2nd edition. Philadelphia: Saunders; 2016: p. 324; with permission.)

extension. In 1 study, Labrador retrievers with hip dysplasia had on average a decrease of 1° hip extension for each year of life.[14] Minor (<10°) loss of joint motion is unlikely to impact limb function, but severe loss of joint motion will likely lead to the dog's inability to gallop, trot, jump up, or climb steps or stairs. It seems to be beneficial, therefore, to assess joint motion in dogs with chronic CHD through the use of goniometric measurements.[9] Because it is much easier to maintain joint motion than to regain it when lost, it seems reasonable to recommend intermittent physical activity that leads to enhanced joint extension (compared with walking on a flat surface) without creating significant clinical signs. Passive ROM, active ROM, and stretching can be incorporated into the early phases of rehabilitation for CHD and continued as part of the daily exercise plan. These activities can help to increase flexibility, prevent adhesions, remodel periarticular fibrosis, and improve extensibility.[15] Passive ROM is completed without muscle contraction by moving the joint through its full ROM. Any additional force applied at the end of the ROM and held for at least a few seconds is defined as stretching. If regaining joint motion is deemed important, a stretching program should be implemented. Stretching is more effective when tissues are heated immediately before and during the stretching session. Passive and active

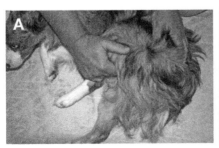
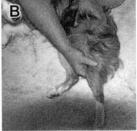

Fig. 3. Passive range of motion to the hip is completed by supporting the femur in 1 hand and the pelvis in the other. (*A*) Hip flexion. (*B*) Hip extension. (*From* Millis D, Levine D. Canine rehabilitation and physical therapy. 2nd edition. Philadelphia: Saunders; 2016. p. 437; with permission.)

ROM in patients with CHD can be beneficial in the early phases of rehabilitation to facilitate appropriate periarticular fibrosis that develops from laxity in younger patients or help to realign fibrous tissue along lines of stress in older patients with clinical OA. Additionally, ROM and stretching can be incorporated into part of the daily exercise program to maintain mobility between soft tissue layers, enhance blood and lymphatic flow, and improve synovial fluid production.[16] Ideally, ROM and stretching are to tissues that are warmed up; therefore, as part of a daily exercise program ROM and stretching can be completed after therapeutic exercises as part of the cool down process. In the early phases of rehabilitation therapy passive ROM and stretching can be performed 2 to 4 times daily for 10 to 20 repetitions. When used as part of the cool down process, ROM and stretching are performed at the end of the exercise program for 15 to 30 repetitions for ROM. For stretching, we empirically recommend performing ten to fifteen 20- to 40-second-long sustained stretches during each session. Sessions may be performed 2 to 3 times per day. With chronic loss of motion, a weekly gain of 3° to 5° of joint motion is anticipated. A thorough explanation of how to perform ROM and stretching exercises is beyond the scope of this article, and can be found elsewhere.[17,18] Joint mobilization may also be incorporated into a rehabilitation program to help increase ROM. Joint mobilization differs from stretching in that when a stretch is applied, a low load is placed on the tissues for a specified amount of time (usually 10–30 seconds) to facilitate elongation. In joint mobilization, the force is applied in an oscillatory manner rather than a sustained manner (**Fig. 4**).

Along with considerations for maintaining and improving joint ROM, proprioception can be affected in patients with OA from chronic CHD. Although little is known about the negative impact of naturally occurring OA on proprioception in dogs, there is clear evidence that OA progresses rapidly in patients with joint injuries that have sensory deficits. In older humans with decreased proprioception, balance exercises readily improve proprioception.[19] In dogs with OA, it is logical to dedicate a small portion of the exercise program to focus on proprioception and balance. In the early phases, this may include weight-shifting exercises (**Fig. 5**) requiring rapid and unpredictable side-to-side weight shifts and, to a lesser extent, front-to-back and back-to-front

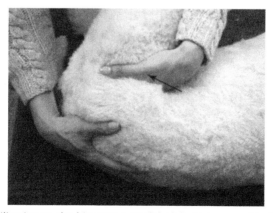

Fig. 4. Joint mobilization to the hip uses a caudal glide to increase hip flexion. The black arrow indicates the direction of the mobilization. (*From* Millis D, Levine D. Canine rehabilitation and physical therapy. 2nd edition. Philadelphia: Saunders; 2016. p. 437; with permission.)

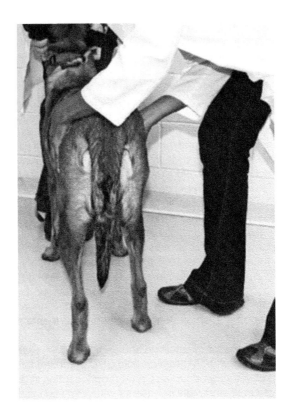

Fig. 5. Weight shifting being applied to the pelvic limbs. This is accomplished by the therapist behind the patient and the hands on either side of the pelvis for support. Pressure is gently applied to 1 side then applied to the other side in a slow, rhythmic fashion. (*From* Millis D, Levine D. Canine rehabilitation and physical therapy. 2nd edition. Philadelphia: Saunders; 2016. p. 487; with permission.)

weight shifts. This is completed by supporting the animal on either side and gently pushing on 1 side, followed by pushing back the other way. The weight-shifting exercises should be done in a slow, rhythmic fashion for 15 to 25 repetitions, 2 to 4 times daily. As balance and proprioception improve, perturbation exercises can be added to the weight shifting with the goal being to disturb the patient's balance just enough for it to recover, but not so much force that the animal falls. Perturbation exercises are performed by gently pushing the animal at the hips without supporting the other side. More complex weight-shifting exercises can be incorporated while the patient is walking to improve dynamic stability. Gently bumping or pushing the animal to 1 side as it is walking to challenge the dog to maintain its balance is 1 way to further improve proprioceptive function.

Additional proprioception and balancing exercises include balance boards, wobble boards, and exercise balls and rolls. A balance board uses a board placed over a fulcrum to rock the dog side to side or forward to backward (**Fig. 6**). A more challenging aspect to balance and proprioception improvement is using a wobble board (**Fig. 7**). Exercise balls and rolls that have been developed for human exercises can be used to improve balance, coordination, and strength. For example, the front limbs can be placed on the ball requiring the dog to maintain static balance of the pelvic

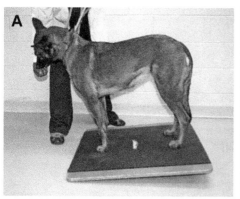
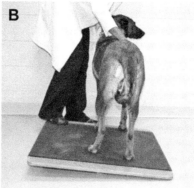

Fig. 6. A balance board is used to provide balance and proprioceptive training (*A*) from the front limbs to the hind limbs and (*B*) from side to side. (*From* Millis D, Levine D. Canine rehabilitation and physical therapy. 2nd edition. Philadelphia: Saunders; 2016. p. 491; with permission.)

limbs (**Fig. 8**). For dynamic challenges, the ball can be rolled forward, backward, and from side to side. This challenges the limbs to maintain balance as movement is occurring. The most challenging use of the exercise balls and rolls is having the patient stand on the therapy ball or roll. This exercise will challenge and engage multiple core stabilizing muscles; therefore, the sessions should be short to avoid fatigue injury.

Other exercises that promote balance and proprioception include standing or walking on foam rubber (**Fig. 9**), mattresses, air mattresses, or trampolines. Furthermore, patients can be walked on various surfaces such as grass, concrete, sand, mulched paths. Altering the texture and evenness of the surface challenges patients' proprioceptive abilities. To facilitate improving balance and proprioception for daily

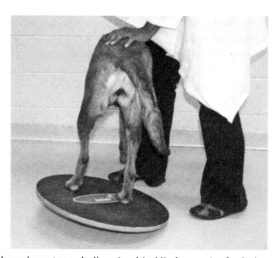

Fig. 7. A wobble board creates a challenging hind limb exercise for balance and proprioceptive training. (*From* Millis D, Levine D. Canine rehabilitation and physical therapy. 2nd edition. Philadelphia: Saunders; 2016. p. 491; with permission.)

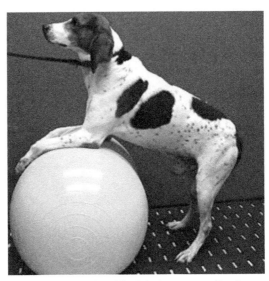

Fig. 8. An exercise ball can improve hind limb balance, coordination, and strength. (*From* Millis D, Levine D. Canine rehabilitation and physical therapy. 2nd edition. Philadelphia: Saunders; 2016. p. 491; with permission.)

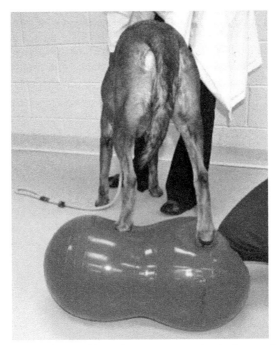

Fig. 9. When walking on foam rubber, the uneven terrain challenges the patient's functional balance and proprioception. (*From* Millis D, Levine D. Canine rehabilitation and physical therapy. 2nd edition. Philadelphia: Saunders; 2016. p. 492; with permission.)

activities, animals should be encouraged to walk over or around obstacles such as low rails, pole weaving, walking on a teeter-totter, and negotiating stairs.

Additional therapeutic exercises that can be incorporated into formal rehabilitation therapy and a home exercise program should be geared toward continued improvement in ROM, specifically in extension of the hip as well as improving weight bearing in a comfortable manner along with building muscle mass and improving muscle fatigue. In structuring a rehabilitation plan for the conservative management of CHD, some basic biomechanics of exercise modification should be understood. Furthermore, the reader is encouraged to learn the biomechanics of physical rehabilitation and kinematics of exercise that can be found elsewhere.[19] The patient should warm up for 5 to 10 minutes before therapeutic exercises.

The simplest of the therapeutic exercises consists of slow, controlled leash walking. Walking can be instituted in the early phases of rehabilitation and can be continued throughout. With regard to the hind limbs, walking will generate approximately 35° of motion in the hip and 40° and 35° of motion in the stifle and hock, respectively.[20,21] Treadmill walking (up to 10° of incline) has been shown to result in the same joint motions as land walking; however, up to 3° of hip extension can be obtained while walking on a inclined (10°) treadmill when compared with walking on land.[19] Although trotting is ideal to increase the speed of muscle contractions and the forces on the limb, it does little to improve ROM in the terms of hip motion compared with walking.[22] Walking up and down stairs or a ramp can facilitate additional flexion and extension to particular joints; however, some consideration has to be placed on the particular exercise for CHD management. For example, incline ramp walking can increase hip flexion by 11%, but does not contribute to improvement in hip extension, which is targeted more commonly in patients with CHD.[23] Walking up stairs is a very good exercise for improving hind limb ROM, such that hip extension can be increased by up to 10° and is greater when compared with walking on level ground (**Fig. 10**).[24] Stair descent results in greater total ROM in the hip (27°) compared with ramp descent (23°).[25]

Having the knowledge of the kinematics of various walking exercises, one is able to create a plan to improve hip ROM as well as improve muscle mass and comfort. For example, in the beginning stages one may use slow controlled leash walking on level ground beginning at 15- to 20-minute intervals 2 to 3 times daily. Once the animal has developed the ability to perform this comfortably, 5 minutes can be added weekly to build up to 30 to 45 minutes. Inclined walking along with stair ascent and descent can be added after several weeks of flat land walking to further improve hip ROM and

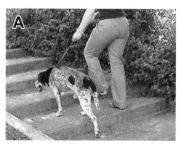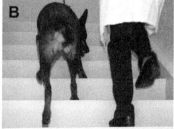

Fig. 10. Walking up stairs to improve hip extension more so than walking on level ground. (*A*) Stairs with a gradual rise. (*B*) Steeper stairs can be used as the patient progresses. (*From* Millis D, Levine D. Canine rehabilitation and physical therapy. 2nd edition. Philadelphia: Saunders; 2016. p. 509; with permission.)

muscle mass. It is also beneficial to add in walking down a declined slope and walking over uneven terrain. Walking on uneven terrain (trail walking, walking through high grass, walking or on sand) forces the patient to increase flexion and extension of various joints to navigate the terrain. All walking exercises should be completed in a stepwise manner, only adding more challenging aspects after the patient has successfully completed easier tasks.

Additional therapeutic exercises such as dancing, Cavaletti rail walking, and sit-to-stand exercises can all help with improving ROM in the hip as part of conservative management for CHD. These exercises can be completed as part of a home exercise program or during formal rehabilitation therapy. Dancing exercises (**Fig. 11**) are designed to increase weight bearing on the rear limbs. This is accomplished by raising the forelimbs off the ground and walking the patient either forward or backward. Interestingly, different kinematics are accomplished by walking the dog forward versus backward. Dancing forward will result in less hip flexion and total hip ROM (22°) compared with walking on level ground (total hip ROM, 33°). Alternatively, dancing backward increases hip extension more than walking on level ground. This difference plays an important role in deciding on what direction dancing exercises should be performed. For example, during the early phases of rehabilitation when hip extension is painful, it may be more comfortable to improve gluteal muscle strengthening by walking the patient forward rather than backward. However, in the later phases when hip extension is improved, walking the patient backward will be more challenging and help to further improve hip extension.[26] Total hip ROM is increased by using Cavaletti rail walking (**Fig. 12**). That increase is proportional to the height of the rails. For example, total hip ROM is improved by 2° (38° total ROM) compared with walking (36° total ROM) with a Cavaletti rail in the low position (level of the carpus). By moving the Cavaletti rail to a medium position total hip ROM is improved to 40° total. In a high position (mid antebrachium) total hip ROM is improved to 43° total. It is

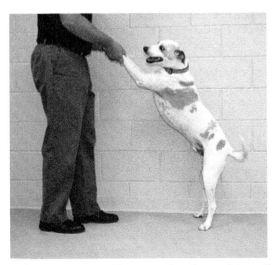

Fig. 11. Dancing exercises to encourage hip range of motion and strength. Initially, dancing the patient forward is less painful and helps to improve gluteal strength. As the patient becomes stronger, dancing the patient backward is more challenging and leads to improved hip extension. (*From* Millis D, Levine D. Canine rehabilitation and physical therapy. 2nd edition. Philadelphia: Saunders; 2016. p. 510; with permission.)

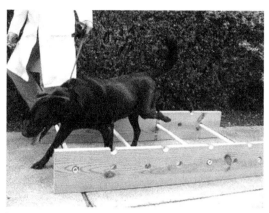

Fig. 12. Example of Cavaletti rail walking to help improve active range of motion (flexion). (*From* Millis D, Levine D. Canine rehabilitation and physical therapy. 2nd edition. Philadelphia: Saunders; 2016. p. 513; with permission.)

important to note that Cavaletti rail walking does not improve joint extension.[27] Sit-to-stand exercises are beneficial in improving both quadriceps and hamstring muscle mass, as well as improving total hip active ROM. Hip extension with sit-to-stand exercises is less compared with walking; however, total hip active ROM is greatly improved (66°) when compared with walking (36°).[28] This is beneficial in the early rehabilitation, when hip extension is still painful, to allow a comfortable exercise that improves overall hip active ROM.

Aquatic therapy has become very versatile in veterinary rehabilitation. It allows active muscle contractions with decreased weight bearing on joints and bones. In patients with CHD, aquatic therapy can help with muscle spasm, muscle weakness, and pain associated with OA. The most significant benefit of aquatic therapy is likely buoyancy, which allows the patient to exercise in an upright position and may decrease pain by minimizing the amount of weight bearing on joints. The higher the water level, the more stress that is taken off of the joints. With water at the level of the lateral malleolus of the fibula, dogs support about 91% of their body weight. With water to the lateral condyle of the femur, dogs support 85% of their body weight. With water to the greater trochanter, dogs are supporting only 38% of their body weight (**Fig. 13**).[29] Another feature of aquatic therapy is hydrostatic pressure and its ability to reduce edema and decrease pain during exercise. This technique is thought to decrease a patient's pain perception, which allows the patient to exercise longer and with less pain.[30] An additional feature of aquatic therapy is the resistance needed to move through the water versus air. This resistance can help to strengthen weak muscles and improve endurance. In patients with OA from associated CHD, underwater treadmill therapy can improve ROM and comfort, while increasing muscular fatigue and building endurance, all while unloading painful joints. Initially, many dogs only tolerate 2 to 5 minutes once or twice weekly. The goal is to work up to 10 to 20 minutes with as few breaks as necessary. Because of the different kinematics of underwater treadmill versus swimming and walking on dry land, in patients with CHD underwater treadmill therapy is likely more beneficial than swimming. Compared with walking on ground, joint flexion is increased in both underwater treadmill walking and swimming; however, almost near normal joint extension is noted in underwater treadmill therapy compared with swimming, where

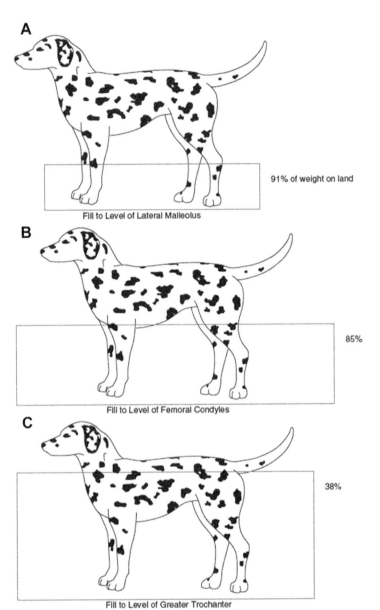

Fig. 13. Amount of body weight borne when immersed in water (*A*) at the height of the lateral malleolus of the fibula, (*B*) to the lateral condyle of the femur, (*C*) at the level of the greater trochanter. Therefore, the higher the water level, the more stress that is taken off of the joints. (*From* Millis D, Levine D. Canine rehabilitation and physical therapy. 2nd edition. Philadelphia: Saunders; 2016. p. 528, with permission; and Levine D, Marcellin-Little DJ, Millis DL, et al. Effects of partial immersion in water on vertical ground reaction forces and weight distribution in dogs. Am J Vet Res 2010;71:1413–16.)

hip joint extension is limited.[31] Furthermore, walking or trotting in the underwater treadmill encourages a more normal gait pattern than swimming. For a more in-depth discussion on the indications, contraindications, parameters, settings, and usages for various physical modalities the reader is encouraged to use additional resources.[32–36]

In summary, dancing backward maximally increases hip extension, whereas sit-to-stand, ramp descent, ramp ascent, and stair descent minimize hip extension. Total hip ROM is maximized with sit-to-stand exercises and dancing forward has the least impact on total hip ROM. Aquatic therapy can further be added to improve muscular strength and endurance as well decrease weight bearing on painful bones and joints. Potential therapeutic exercises used to manage canine CHD are listed in **Table 1**. For more in-depth therapeutic exercises to improve joint motion, strengthen, improve endurance and speed, the reader is encouraged to read additional sources.[37]

Physical Modalities to Improve Range of Motion, Comfort, and Function

Physical modalities can be used in rehabilitation therapy to augment therapeutic exercises and promote tissue healing. Modalities such as therapeutic ultrasound, electrical stimulation, laser therapy, and extracorporeal shockwave therapy (ESWT) can be used to manage CHD. Therapeutic ultrasound can be beneficial to patients with OA associated with CHD by improving ROM and decreasing pain and muscle spasm. It allows heating of deeper tissues than cannot be reached with hot packing. Therapeutic ultrasound depth penetration changes based on frequency: 1.0 MHz heats to a depth ranging from 2 to 5 cm and 3.3 MHz heats from 0.5 to 3 cm.[38] Hot packing can heat tissue up to 2 cm; however, the greatest temperature change is noted from the skin surface to approximately 1 cm in depth. The thermal effect of therapeutic ultrasound may increase collagen extensibility, blood flow, pain threshold, and enzyme activity. Therapeutic ultrasound can be incorporated into a rehabilitation protocol in the management of CHD to heat the tissues to further improve stretching and ROM for maximal benefit. To achieve this an intensity of 1.0 to 2.0 W/cm^2 could be used with either 1.0 or 3.3 MHz frequencies, depending on dog breed and size. Treatment time varies, but is typically 8 to 10 minutes. The thermal effects of therapeutic ultrasound are short lived. Therefore, ROM and stretching exercises should occur while the tissue is heated or immediately afterward.

Electrical stimulation increases muscle strength and ROM, improves muscle tone, improves pain control, and decreases edema and muscle spasm.[39] Neuromuscular electrical stimulation is used for muscle reeducation, prevention of muscle atrophy,

Table 1	
Therapeutic exercises potentially included in the management of canine hip dysplasia	
Purpose	**Possible Therapeutic Exercises**
Increasing limb strength	Daily walk or trot >10 min; tunnel walk, sit to stand, and stand to sit repetitions, swimming
Increasing core strength	Daily walk or trot >10 min; swimming
Increasing cardiovascular fitness	Daily walk or trot >10 min
Stretching pelvic limbs	Climbing up slopes, hills, and stairs; low jumps
Increasing proprioception	Daily walk or trot >10 min; walk on soft surfaces: sand, mulch, gravel, leaves, grass; teeter-totter or pole weaving

and enhanced joint movement, whereas transcutaneous electrical nerve stimulation is commonly used for pain control. In patients with CHD, electrical stimulation can be incorporated into a rehabilitation program to help with long-standing muscle atrophy or selected strengthening of muscle groups (hamstrings, gluteals, or quadriceps) by using neuromuscular electrical stimulation twice weekly for 10 to 20 minutes. In patients with chronic OA pain associated with CHD, transcutaneous electrical nerve stimulation can be used for relief of pain. Treatment can be 2 to 3 times weekly for 30 minutes.

Laser therapy can be used to relieve pain, reduce inflammation, and increase microcirculation through the concept of photobiomodulation. The antiinflammatory and analgesic benefit of laser therapy for patients with OA has been described.[40–42] For patients with OA from CHD, 8 to 10 J/cm^2 are used and the entire hip area is treated. Start treatment at the greater trochanter, then direct the probe head around the cranial, medial, and caudal surfaces of the hip in a circumferential pattern. Because of compensatory changes, referred pain from the lumbosacral and epaxial areas can be treated as well. Treatment protocols vary, but initially 6 treatments are applied over 3 weeks, followed by maintenance treatments every 3 to 4 weeks. Regardless of the treatment protocol, the treatment is designed to achieve the appropriate dose, number of treatments, and interval between treatments.

The use of ESWT is centered around the pain-relieving response in patients with OA from chronic CHD. Shock waves are acoustic waves with various frequencies that are delivered and travel through soft tissues to the target area. Once the shockwave reaches the target, energy is then released, which creates a biologic response promoting analgesia and decreasing certain inflammatory mediators. The analgesic effect after ESWT is poorly understood, but thought to be due to the release of cytokines and growth factors centered around decreasing inflammation and swelling. In dogs with hip OA, ESWT improved ground reaction forces after 4 weeks of treatment, and benefits lasted as long as 3 months.[43] In a human study of arthritic chondrocytes, inflammatory factors (tumor necrosis factor-alpha and interleukin-10) were found to be decreased in patients treated with ESWT when compared with the pretreated chondrocytes.[44] The effects of ESWT on articular cartilage is an area of concern that warrants additional investigation because preliminary research suggests that high-energy ESWT applied directly to cartilage may cause degenerative changes.[45,46] Patients are sedated or anesthetized before ESWT. Typically, 500 to 1000 shocks are applied with an energy level of 0.15 mJ/mm^2 and 180 pulses/min to the hip region for 2 treatments spaced 3 to 4 weeks apart. Improvement may be noted for days to several months after treatment.

Selecting a Treatment Program for a Conservative Approach to Canine Hip Dysplasia

Arthritic dogs with minor locomotion problems will have a treatment program focused on decreasing pain, maintaining optimal weight, maintaining limb and core strength, stretching affected joints, and stimulating proprioception. Pain management is generally achieved with simple pharmacologic steps, rest, and exercise supervision and customization. Pharmacologic and other forms of pain relief may be intermittent as long as dogs adhere to a long-term exercise program. Because OA screening is not done routinely in dogs, OA is most often discovered in its later stages. Losing mobility because of severe OA is common in large breed dogs. For patients with severe OA, it is important to implement all possible support strategies to decrease the impact of the disease on the dogs' well-being and mobility. These may include multimodal pharmacologic management, ice, heat, massage, acupuncture, acupressure, electroacupuncture, transcutaneous electrical nerve stimulation, and rest. Once pain is managed, it is important to initiate an initially conservative and subsequently progressive exercise program. Patients with severe OA may need temporary or permanent ambulation assistance. Slings are the most common and cost-effective ambulation assistance devices. Severely impaired dogs may benefit from an ambulation cart. Underwater treadmills significantly reduce pelvic limb peak vertical force[30] and are useful in building muscle in a weight-minimized environment. Overall, a management program for companion animals with OA should be simple and logical. Managing pain is the first priority for all patients. The program must then address the most critical aspects of each patient's unique situation and, over time, improve the patient's mobility, strength, proprioception and, above all, quality of life.

PHYSICAL REHABILITATION AFTER SURGICAL MANAGEMENT OF HIP DYSPLASIA

Surgical intervention is recommended in older patients with debilitating OA that have failed medical, conservative, and rehabilitative therapies or in younger patients to provide a good, pain-free quality of life. The type of surgical intervention is dictated by the clinical signs present, age, and if the clinical signs of CHD are owing to underlying laxity in the early phases or secondary OA in the later phases. Rehabilitation therapy is paramount and in the authors' opinion considered the standard of care after surgery for CHD. Rehabilitation therapy will improve overall comfort, ROM, early usage of the postoperative limb, and facilitate healing.

Rehabilitation Therapy After Juvenile Pubic Symphysiodesis

The fusion of the medial growth plates of the pubis, referred to as juvenile pubic symphysiodesis (JPS) is sometimes performed in dogs around the age of 16 weeks with the intent to alter pelvic growth to increase dorsal coverage of the femoral head. Dogs undergo JPS to control hip subluxation.[47] Subluxation persists after surgery, but altered growth of the pubis increases the dorsal coverage of the femoral head by the dorsal acetabular rim. Tissue trauma after a JPS is relatively minor and does not warrant specific rehabilitation strategies to accelerate the resorption of edema or decrease focal pain. Also, the strength of the pelvis is not compromised after a JPS, unlike after a double or triple pelvic osteotomy, where the ilium is osteotomized and stabilized with a bone plate. The key aim of rehabilitation after JPS is to minimize the impact of hip subluxation during skeletal development. Dogs with hip subluxation will benefit from having strong muscles around the hip (gluteal muscles, pectineus, adductor, rectus femoris, etc). Growth optimization is also critical: large breed puppies should not be eating ad libitum (as much as they want to eat), they should not overeat carbohydrates, and they should not receive calcium or phosphorus supplementation. The primary focus of rehabilitation is to promote muscular development of the hind limbs with low-impact exercises.

Rehabilitation Therapy After Triple or Double Pelvic Osteotomy

Triple or double pelvic osteotomies are performed on dogs that have early clinical signs of CHD but have not progressed to the point of having significant radiographic evidence of OA. Most dogs that fit these criteria are between 4 and 10 months of age.[5] When performed, the triple pelvic osteotomy or double pelvic osteotomy, much like a JPS will improve dorsal femoral head coverage. The technique involves making 2 or 3 osteotomies: one in the pubis, one in the ischium (only in triple pelvic osteotomy), and one in the ilium. The caudal ileal segment is variably rotated, based on the amount of subluxation; rotation is commonly 20°. A bone plate is applied to stabilize the ileal osteotomy.[5]

Rehabilitation initially includes specific activity supervision for 4 to 6 weeks to allow bone healing. During this time, nonsteroidal antiinflammatory drugs, cryotherapy, and passive ROM are used to maintain and normalize hip motion. Controlled, low-impact therapeutic exercises, such as sit-to-stand exercises, and aquatic walking may be useful to attenuate muscle atrophy while avoiding excessive stress on the repair. Muscle strengthening can be achieved using controlled walking, aquatic walking, and low-impact exercises. The duration of these activities is increased gradually during the first 3 months. Dogs are restricted to leash walking, with no running or jumping for the first 3 months to reduce the chances of implant loosening or hip luxation.

Rehabilitation Therapy After Femoral Head and Neck Ostectomy

Rehabilitation after femoral head and neck ostectomy emphasizes gaining hip extension, muscle mass, and active use of the pelvic limb. In the authors' opinion, rehabilitation should imperatively begin within 48 hours after femoral head and neck ostectomy and continue until normal weight bearing is achieved on the surgical limb. A sample rehabilitation protocol is included in Appendix A.

After surgery, nonsteroidal antiinflammatory drugs, cryotherapy, and hip passive ROM (especially for hip extension) should be performed daily. In addition to passive ROM for hip extension, ambulation on land, a ground treadmill, or an underwater treadmill can be used to promote active hip extension and weight bearing. Walking up inclines will emphasize strengthening of the hip extensor muscle groups. Dancing exercises encourage muscle strengthening and improve hip ROM, especially in extension. Most dogs will toe touch consistently within 1 to 2 weeks, bear partial weight in 3 weeks, and be actively using the leg by 4 weeks. Deep heating (up to 5 cm) may be accomplished by the use of therapeutic ultrasound,[48] and may be performed before stretching. The animal should regain near-normal walking and trotting gaits, but full ROM is rarely achieved, with hip extension being the most limited. Prognosis for return to daily function is good, but varies with the chronicity of the preexisting lameness and the presence of comorbidities. The dog's overall athletic ability will likely be decreased. Large dogs tend to have more difficulty with recovery than small dogs, and unfit and obese dogs tend to have more difficulty than fit and athletic dogs.

Rehabilitation Therapy After Total Hip Arthroplasty/Replacement

Total hip replacement (THR) is a well-established management option for dogs with severe CHD. THR is generally delayed until CHD can no longer be managed by the use of medical therapy and exercise.

Rehabilitation after THR can be divided into conventional rehabilitation, performed in uncomplicated patients, and targeted rehabilitation, performed to address specific situations relating to THR.

General rehabilitation after total hip replacement

The goal of rehabilitation after THR is to restore the long-term, pain-free use of the operated limb.[49] Several retrospective and a few prospective studies of canine THR have been published.[50–52] These studies included little information regarding postoperative rehabilitation beyond initial supportive care and progressive leash walks. In a long-term prospective clinical trial in which physical rehabilitation was limited to walking dogs on a leash to void during the first 2 months after surgery and increasing the length of leash walks during weeks 9 to 12, hip passive ROM was normal in 29 of 31 dogs (94%) that were free of complications 5 years after surgery.[52] Hip extension was decreased in 3 dogs with long-term implant luxation and in 1 dog with a femoral osteosarcoma. In the same study, thigh girth was equal to or greater than the opposite thigh in all dogs that were complication free. To our knowledge, there are no published reports describing dogs that did not achieve proper limb function after THR, provided that the hips were free of implant malposition, infection, fracture, or failure of fracture fixation. Functionally, dogs undergoing routine THR have normal limb use 3 months after surgery.[51] This suggests that specific rehabilitation programs or long hospitalization periods are probably not necessary for the success of uncomplicated THRs, but they may be considered in patients with limited hip motion because of tissue tightness. For example, some patients with dorsal femoral displacement for extended periods before surgery have tight periarticular muscles and other soft tissues after joint replacement.

Rehabilitation includes acute, subacute, and chronic phases. Acutely, the rehabilitation after THR is focused on providing pain relief, and avoiding catastrophic complications, including implant luxation or femoral, fracture. Subacute rehabilitation after THR is focused on completing the recovery of joint motion and strengthening of the operated and contralateral limbs. Because healing is still progressing, exercises that would place excessive stress on the joint capsule and bone–implant interfaces are avoided. Excessive stress on the joint capsule could result from external rotation, from excessive adduction, or from excessive abduction of the operated limb. Walking exercises are generally performed in a straight line. Slippery and unsteady surfaces are avoided.

Chronic rehabilitation after THR is focused on strengthening the operated and contralateral limbs. A wider range of therapeutic exercises is introduced and the intensity of these exercises increases over time (**Fig. 14**).

Targeted rehabilitation after total hip replacement

Tissue tension Dogs with limited hip extension will benefit from a stretching program. When the loss of hip extension is severe, moist heat and manual stretching techniques are used. Extension uses a spinning motion of the femoral head on the acetabulum and thus tightens the joint capsule at end ranges. This is a safe direction for stretching with regard to limiting the possibility for luxating the hip with overzealous motion, but care must be exercised to not cause the patient pain with this stretch. After the stretching session, active hip extension exercises should be performed to retrain the patient to use increased ROM. Manual stretching is not critical when the loss of hip extension is modest and the patient's limb use is acceptable. Some patients are not receptive to stretching techniques and owners may not be able to safely perform stretching at home. In these situations, targeted therapeutic exercises alone can be used instead to gain hip extension for a more normal gait pattern and better function. Walking up a gentle incline, stepping up a single step or a series of steps with adequate traction, and stepping over objects all place the trailing limb in increased hip extension.

Sciatic neurapraxia Patients with sciatic neurapraxia typically present with knuckling and weakness of the muscles in the sciatic distribution, including the hamstrings and crus musculature. Dogs exhibiting deficits owing to sciatic neurapraxia after

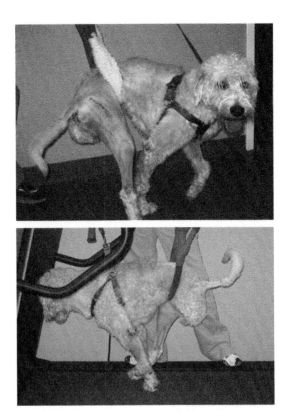

Fig. 14. Example of a patient walking on a land treadmill after a total hip replacement for severe canine hip dysplasia. This patient had previously had a contralateral mid-femoral amputation. Note the sling being used to support the pelvic limb so the patient cannot slip or fall during the exercise session. (*From* Marcellin-Little DJ, Doyle ND, Pyke JF. Physical rehabilitation after total joint arthroplasty in companion animals. Vet Clin North Am Small Anim Pract 2015;45(1):151; with permission.)

THR need rehabilitation for days to months, depending on the severity of the deficits.[53] Rehabilitation focuses on minimizing hip complications owing to decreased active muscular stabilization and protection (such as luxation), avoiding skin abrasions resulting from scuffing or knuckling, decreasing the loss of muscle mass in muscles innervated by branches of the sciatic nerve, and strengthening the affected muscle groups. Neuromuscular electrical stimulation can be used to elicit muscle contractions of the affected muscles to attenuate atrophy,[33] but is not universally well-accepted by patients. If active hock extension is absent for weight bearing, the hock can be stabilized by an orthosis during therapeutic exercises (**Fig. 15**). Once hock extension improves, the dog can exercise without an orthosis.[54] To avoid abrasions, affected dogs should avoid walking on abrasive surfaces and metacarpals and toes should be protected by a thin bootie or bandage. If the patient frequently knuckles, bootie systems with support straps that pull the hock into flexion and the digits into extension (TheraPaw, Lebanon, NJ) can be used during ambulation and therapeutic exercise sessions to create a more normal posture for functional limb use while simultaneously protecting the skin from abrasions. In dogs with weak hock flexion, an exercise band or rubber traction band (Anti-

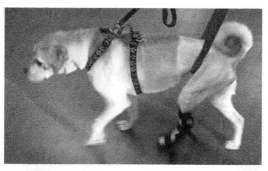

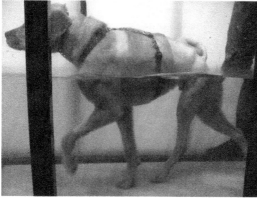

Fig. 15. A patient with sciatic neurapraxia after a total hip replacement. In the upper image, the patient is wearing a tarsal orthotic, which will allow the patient to exercise without scuffing or knuckling while walking. Use of underwater treadmill therapy allows the patient to exercise without scuffing or knuckling. (*From* Marcellin-Little DJ, Doyle ND, Pyke JF. Physical rehabilitation after total joint arthroplasty in companion animals. Vet Clin North Am Small Anim Pract 2015;45(1):159; with permission.)

Knuckling Device; Canine Mobility, Seattle, WA; or Biko Mobility, Raleigh, NC) can be used to facilitate more normal flexion ROM during exercises. Exercises to strengthen hock flexion include stepping over progressively taller objects, such as segments of PVC pipe, walking in water at the height of the hock, and elicitation of a flexor withdraw reflex by pinching the digits. Most dogs fully recover from sciatic neurapraxia.[53]

Implant luxation (dorsal/ventral) After the acute management of a luxation, either traumatic or after a THR (with reduction/hobbles and/or surgical revision), targeted strengthening of the appropriate muscle groups provides improved dynamic joint support to help prevent a recurrence. Dogs that experienced a dorsal luxation need additional strengthening of the muscles lying on the dorsal aspect of the hip. Suggested exercises include 3-legged standing (lifting the unaffected pelvic limb and cuing the dog to shift weight onto the operative limb while maintaining a level pelvis), balancing on a soft or unsteady surface (commercial balance discs or an air mattress), walking perpendicular to an incline with the operative limb "downhill," and the previously mentioned hip extension exercises. Dogs experiencing a ventral luxation require strengthening of the adductors. Suggested exercises include resisted TheraBand exercises (TheraBand, Akron, OH) while walking on a treadmill or alongside the handler (pull the hip into abduction with the band wrapped around the thigh to stimulate a contraction of the adductors), walking sideways, or walking perpendicular to an incline with the operative limb "uphill." Underwater treadmill walking also can effectively and safely target the desired muscle group in both situations,[58] particularly in the earlier phases of recovery. Proprioceptive retraining should also be used to improve body awareness and coordination for decreased risk of future falls.

SUMMARY

The goals of rehabilitation therapy at various stages of CHD vary. Initially, clinical signs and discomfort are thought to be owing to the underlying laxity. This laxity results in lateralization of the femoral head during the swing phase of the gait with a "catastrophic reduction" of the femoral head into the acetabulum during foot strike. Rehabilitation therapy as part of conservative management in patients with laxity or in older patients with OA is centered around maintaining pain control and comfort while improving hip ROM in extension and maintenance of muscle mass. This is accomplished with weight reduction and fitness, minimizing joint pain, pharmaceuticals, disease-modifying osteoarthritic agents, manual therapies, therapeutic exercises, and physical modalities. Surgical therapy for patients with CHD is focused at improving femoral head coverage and reducing the development of OA (JPS, triple pelvic osteotomy/double pelvic osteotomy) or removing the source of discomfort (femoral head and neck ostectomy or THR). Initially, rehabilitation therapy is designed to improve overall postoperative comfort, ROM, early use of the postoperative limb, and facilitate healing. The later stages of rehabilitation therapy are continuation of improvement in ROM and muscle mass to facilitate return to function once surgical healing is satisfactory. Each aspect of rehabilitation such as manual, therapeutic, and physical modalities follows a multimodal patient centered approach.

REFERENCES

1. Johnson JA, Austin C, Breur GJ. Incidence of canine appendicular musculoskeletal disorders in 16 veterinary teaching hospitals from 1980-1989. Vet Comp Orthop Traumatol 1994;7:56–69.
2. Riser WH. The dog as a model for the study of hip dysplasia. Growth, form, and development of the normal and dysplastic hip joint. Vet Pathol 1975;12:234–334.
3. Paster ER, LaFond E, Biery DN, et al. Estimates of prevalence of hip dysplasia in Golden Retrievers and Rottweilers and the influence of bias on published prevalence figures. J Am Vet Med Assoc 2005;226:387–92.
4. Smith GK, Karbe GT, Agnello KA, et al. Pathogenesis, diagnosis, and control of canine hip dysplasia. In: Tobias KM, Johnston SA, editors. Veterinary surgery, small animal. 1st edition. St Louis (MO): Elsevier Saunders; 2012. p. 824–48.
5. Roush JK. Surgical therapy of canine hip dysplasia. In: Tobias KM, Johnston SA, editors. Veterinary surgery, small animal. 1st edition. St Louis (MO): Elsevier Saunders; 2012. p. 849–64.
6. Davidson JR, Kerwin S. Common orthopedic conditions and their physical rehabilitation. In: Millis DL, Levine D, editors. Canine rehabilitation and physical therapy. 2nd edition. Philadelphia: Elsevier Saunders; 2014. p. 543–81.
7. Smith GK, Paster ER, Powers MY, et al. Lifelong diet restriction and radiographic evidence of osteoarthritis of the hip joint in dogs. J Am Vet Med Assoc 2006;229:690–3.

8. Jaegger G, Marcellin-Little DJ, Levine D. Reliability of goniometry in Labrador Retrievers. Am J Vet Res 2002;63:979–86.
9. Millis DL, Levine D. The role of exercise and physical modalities in the treatment of osteoarthritis. Vet Clin North Am Small Anim Pract 1997;27:913–30.
10. Millard RP, Towle-Millard HA, Rankin DC, et al. Effect of cold compress application on tissue temperature in healthy dogs. Am J Vet Res 2013;74:443–7.
11. Oosterveld FG, Rasker JJ. Treating arthritis with locally applied heat or cold. Semin Arthritis Rheum 1994;24:82–90.
12. Danneskiold-Samsoe B, Bartels EM. Massage-is it really a reliable method of treatment? Eur J Pain 1999;3:244–5.
13. Millard RP, Towle-Millard HA, Rankin DC, et al. Effect of warm compress application on tissue temperature in healthy dogs. Am J Vet Res 2013;74:448–51.
14. Greene LM, Marcellin-Little DJ, Lascelles BD. Associations among exercise duration, lameness severity, and hip joint range of motion in Labrador Retrievers with hip dysplasia. J Am Vet Med Assoc 2013;242:1528–33.
15. Millis DL, Levine D. Range-of-motion and stretching exercises. In: Millis DL, Levine D, editors. Canine rehabilitation and physical therapy. 2nd edition. Philadelphia: Elsevier Saunders; 2014. p. 431–46.
16. Brody LT. Mobility impairment. In: Hall CM, Brody LT, editors. Therapeutic exercise: moving toward function. Philadelphia: Lippincott Williams & Wilkins; 1999. p. 87–111.
17. Westlake KP, Wu Y, Culham EG. Sensory-specific balance training in older adults: effect on position, movement, and velocity sense at the ankle. Phys Ther 2007;87: 560–8.
18. Saunders DG, Walker JR, Levine D. Joint mobilization. Vet Clin North Am Small Anim Pract 2005;35:1287–316.
19. Weigel JP, Arnold G, Hicks DA, et al. Biomechanics of rehabilitation. Vet Clin North Am Small Anim Pract 2005;35:1255–85.
20. Hottinger HA, DeCamp CE, Olivier NB, et al. Noninvasive kinematic analysis of the walk in healthy large-breed dogs. Am J Vet Res 1996;57:381–8.
21. DeCamp CE, Riggs CM, Olivier NB, et al. Kinematic evaluation of gait in dogs with cranial cruciate ligament rupture. Am J Vet Res 1996;57:120–6.
22. DeCamp CE, Soutas-Little RW, Hauptman J, et al. Kinematic gait analysis of the trot in healthy greyhounds. Am J Vet Res 1993;54:627–34.
23. Holler PJ, Brazda V, Dal-Bianco B, et al. Kinematic motion analysis of the joints of the forelimbs and hind limbs of dogs during walking exercise regimens. Am J Vet Res 2010;71:734–40.
24. Durant AM, Millis DL, Headrick JF. Kinematics of stair ascent in healthy dogs. Vet Comp Orthop Traumatol 2011;24:99–105.
25. Richards J, Holler P, Bockstahler B, et al. A comparison of human and canine kinematics during level walking, stair ascent, and stair descent. Wien Tierärtz Mschr 2010;97:92–100.
26. Millis DL, Schwartz P, Hicks DA, et al. Kinematic assessment of selected therapeutic exercises in dogs. In: 3rd International Symposium on Physical Therapy and Rehabilitation in Veterinary Medicine. Raleigh, NC, August 2004.
27. Headrick JH, Hicks DA, McEachern GL. Kinematics of walking over Cavaletti rails compared with over ground walking in dogs. In: 2nd World Veterinary Orthopedic Congress Veterinary Orthopedic Society. Keystone, CO, February/March 2006.
28. Feeney LC, Lin CF, Marcellin-Little DJ, et al. Validation of two-dimensional kinematic analysis of walk and sit-to-stand motions in dogs. Am J Vet Res 2007;68: 277–82.

29. Levine D, Marcellin-Little DJ, Millis DL, et al. Effects of partial immersion in water on vertical ground reaction forces and weight distribution in dogs. Am J Vet Res 2010;71:1413–6.

30. Johns KM. Aquatic therapy: therapeutic treatment for today's patient. Phys Ther Prod 1993;24–5.

31. Marsolais GS, McLean S, Derrick T, et al. Kinematic analysis of the hind limb during swimming and walking in healthy dogs and dogs with surgically corrected cranial cruciate ligament rupture. J Am Vet Med Assoc 2003;222:739–43.

32. Levine D, Watson T. Therapeutic ultrasound. In: Millis DL, Levine D, editors. Canine rehabilitation and physical therapy. Philadelphia: Elsevier Saunders; 2014. p. 328–41.

33. Levine D, Bockstahler B. Electrical stimulation. In: Millis DL, Levine D, editors. Canine rehabilitation and physical therapy. Philadelphia: Elsevier Saunders; 2014. p. 342–58.

34. Pryor B, Millis DL. Therapeutic laser in veterinary medicine. Vet Clin North Am Small Anim Pract 2015;45:45–56.

35. Durant A, Millis DL. Applications of extracorporeal shockwave in small animal rehabilitation. In: Millis DL, Levine D, editors. Canine rehabilitation and physical therapy. 2nd edition. Philadelphia: Elsevier Saunders; 2014. p. 381–92.

36. Levine D, Millis DL, Flocker J, et al. Aquatic therapy. In: Millis DL, Levine D, editors. Canine rehabilitation and physical therapy. 2nd edition. Philadelphia: Elsevier Saunders; 2014. p. 526–42.

37. Millis DL, Drum M, Levine D. Therapeutic exercises: joint motion, strengthening, endurance, and speed exercises. In: Millis DL, Levine D, editors. Canine rehabilitation and physical therapy. 2nd edition. Philadelphia: Elsevier Saunders; 2014. p. 506–25.

38. Shulthies SS. Interview with Dr. David O Draper. Sports Phys Ther Sect Newslett Am Phys Ther Assoc 1995;12–3.

39. Nelson RM, Hayes KW, Currier DP. Clinical electrotherapy. 3rd edition. Norwalk (CT): Appleton & Lange; 1999.

40. de Morais NC, Barbosa AM, Vale ML, et al. Anti-inflammatory effect of low-level laser and light-emitting diode in zymosan-induced arthritis. Photomed Laser Surg 2010;28:227–32.

41. Rubio CR, Cremonezzi D, Moya M, et al. Helium-neon laser reduces the inflammatory process of arthritis. Photomed Laser Surg 2010;28:125–9.

42. Brosseau L, Robinson V, Wells G, et al. Low level laser therapy (Classes I, II and III) for treating rheumatoid arthritis. Cochrane Database Syst Rev 2005;(4):CD002049.

43. Mueller M, Bockstahler B, Skalicky M, et al. Effects of radial shockwave therapy on the limb function of dogs with hip osteoarthritis. Vet Rec 2007;160:762–5.

44. Moretti B, Iannone F, Notarnicola A, et al. Extracorporeal shock waves downregulate the expression of interleukin-10 and tumor necrosis factor-alpha in osteoarthritic chondrocytes. BMC Musculoskelet Disord 2008;9:16.

45. Dorotka R, Kubista B, Schatz KD, et al. Effects of extracorporeal shock waves on human articular chondrocytes and ovine bone marrow stromal cells in vitro. Arch Orthop Trauma Surg 2003;123:345–8.

46. Mayer-Wagner S, Ernst J, Maier M, et al. The effect of high-energy extracorporeal shock waves on hyaline cartilage of adult rats in vivo. J Orthop Res 2010;28:1050–6.

47. Dueland RT, Adams WM, Fialkowski JP, et al. Effects of pubic symphysiodesis in dysplastic puppies. Vet Surg 2001;30:201–17.

48. Levine D, Millis DL, Mynatt T. Effects of 3.3-MHz ultrasound on caudal thigh muscle temperature in dogs. Vet Surg 2001;30:170–4.

49. Marcellin-Little DJ, Doyle ND, Pyke JF. Physical rehabilitation after total joint arthroplasty in companion animals. Vet Clin North Am Small Anim Pract 2015;45: 145–65.

50. Peck J, Liska W, DeYoung D, et al. Clinical application of total hip replacement. In: Peck J, Marcellin-Little D, editors. Advances in small animal total joint replacement. 1st edition. Ames (IA): Wiley-Blackwell; 2013.

51. Lascelles BD, Freire M, Roe SC, et al. Evaluation of functional outcome after BFX total hip replacement using a pressure sensitive walkway. Vet Surg 2010;39:71–7.

52. Marcellin-Little DJ, DeYoung BA, Doyens DH, et al. Canine uncemented porous-coated anatomic total hip arthroplasty: results of a long-term prospective evaluation of 50 consecutive cases. Vet Surg 1999;28:10–20.

53. Andrews CM, Liska WD, Roberts DJ. Sciatic neurapraxia as a complication in 1000 consecutive canine total hip replacements. Vet Surg 2008;37:254–62.

54. Levine JM, Fitch RB. Use of an ankle-foot orthosis in a dog with traumatic sciatic neuropathy. J Small Anim Pract 2003;44:236–8.

APPENDIX A: SAMPLE PROTOCOL FOR FEMORAL HEAD AND NECK OSTECTOMY

Phase	Expected Timeframe[a]	Rehabilitation Clinic Program	Home Program	Outcome Assessment Measures	Criteria for Movement to Next Phase
Non–weight bearing to toe-touching	Immediate to 48–72 h postoperative	Therapeutic exercises Slow, gentle hip pROM for operated limb focusing on extension (10 reps TID-QID beginning immediately postoperative while recovering from anesthesia) Slow leash walking with sling support available, only to go outside (up to 5 min, TID-QID) Balance exercises on a soft foam pad or bidirectional balance board for weight bearing Modalities Gentle massage around the surgery site, thigh and lumbosacral regions Transcutaneous electrical stimulation for pain relief (15–20 min SID-TID) Cryotherapy (15–20 min TID after activities) – *first session immediately postoperative in combination with slow pROM while recovering from anesthesia* Therapeutic laser therapy SID	Inpatient status preferred during this phase If home: Therapeutic exercises Slow, gentle hip pROM for operated limb focusing on extension (10 reps TID-QID beginning immediately postoperative) Slow leash walking with sling support available, only to go outside (up to 5 min, TID-QID) Balance exercises on a semifirm surface for weight bearing Modalities Gentle massage around the surgery site, thigh and lumbosacral regions Cryotherapy (15–20 min TID after activities) – *first session immediately postoperative*	Postoperative bilateral "hip" pROM and other joints as applicable via goniometry Postoperative bilateral thigh circumference Response to activity and subjective pain level Lameness score at a stance and walk Weight	Early toe-touching Adequate resting analgesia Decreased perioperative swelling and lack of incisional drainage.

| Early weight bearing | 72 h to 2 weeks postoperative | Therapeutic exercises pROM and flexion/extension hip stretches of operated limb (10–15 reps BID-TID). Bicycling and flexor reflex exercises Slow, controlled walking on a land treadmill, 5–10 min including mild incline settings to encourage hip extension and target gluteal muscles Balance exercises on a soft foam pad or bidirectional balance board for weight bearing BID-TID Modalities Heat therapy before activity (10–15 min BID-TID, not within 72 h after surgery or if S/S of acute inflammation are still present) Therapeutic ultrasound SID Massage Therapeutic laser therapy PRN Cryotherapy (15–20 min BID) after exercises | Therapeutic exercises pROM and flexion/extension hip stretches of operated limb (10–15 reps BID-TID) Slow, controlled leash walking, 5–20 min including mild inclines to encourage hip extension and target gluteal muscles Balance exercises on a soft foam pad for weight bearing BID-TID Modalities Heat therapy (10–15 min BID-TID, before exercises, Not within 72 h after surgery or if clinical signs of acute inflammation are still present) Cryotherapy (15–20 min BID) after exercises | Goniometry - hip ROM and other joints if applicable Response to activity and subjective pain level Lameness score at a stance and walk Weight | Consistent partial weight bearing on operated limb on all strides at a walk Minimal pain with light activities Incisional healing without complications |

(continued on next page)

(continued)

Phase	Expected Timeframe[a]	Rehabilitation Clinic Program	Home Program	Outcome Assessment Measures	Criteria for Movement to Next Phase
Consistent weight bearing at walk	2–4 wk postoperative	Therapeutic exercises pROM and flexion/extension hip stretches of operated limb (10–15 reps SID-BID Controlled walking on a land treadmill, 10–15 min with increased incline angle and speed SID Balance exercises on an inflatable disk or 360° wobble board for weight bearing 5 min BID-TID Encourage increased weight bearing on operated limb (examples: initiating dancing exercises as tolerated 5 min BID-TID, applying weight on operated limb at 3%–5% body weight or syringe cap under contralateral foot) Sit-to-stand exercises 5–10 reps BID Aquatic therapy: UWTM walking 5–10 min once incision is sealed SID-BID Swimming 3–5 d per week Cavaletti Rails 5–10 reps BID Modalities Heat therapy before activity Therapeutic ultrasound PRN Massage PRN Therapeutic laser therapy PRN Cryotherapy (15–20 min BID) after exercises	Therapeutic exercises pROM and flexion/extension hip stretches of operated limb (10–15 reps BID-TID) Leash walks 15–20 min including 5–10 min of inclines Balance exercises on an inflatable disk for weight bearing BID-TID Sit-to-stand exercises 5–10 reps BID Light jogging 3–5 min per day Stairs: 1 flight SID-BID Modalities Heat therapy (10 min) before activity Cryotherapy (15–20 min) after exercises	Goniometry - hip ROM and other joints if applicable Reevaluate thigh muscle girth at 3–4 wk postoperative Response to activity and subjective pain level Lameness score at a stance, walk and trot Weight	Consistent weight bearing on operated limb on all strides at a walk, consistent partial weight bearing at a trot Minimal pain with light activities

Consistent weight bearing at a trot	5–8 wk postoperative	Therapeutic exercises	Therapeutic exercises	Goniometry - hip ROM and other joints if applicable	Consistent weight bearing on operated limb at a trot
		pROM and flexion/extension hip stretches of operated limb PRN	pROM and flexion/ extension hip stretches of operated limb PRN	Reevaluate thigh muscle girth at 7–8 wk postoperative	Minimal to no pain with moderate to extensive activities
		Controlled walking or light jogging on a land treadmill, 15–20 min with increased incline angle and speed SID	Leash walks 20–30 min including up to 10–15 min of inclines, may use weights on affected limb or pulled with a harness as tolerated/required	Response to activity and subjective pain level	
		Balance exercises on an inflatable disk or 360° wobble board for weight bearing 10 min BID-TID	Incorporate challenging surfaces to walks that is, snow, sand, when possible	Lameness score at a stance, walk and trot	
		Sit-to-stand exercises 10–20 reps BID	Controlled ball-playing with gradually increasing times and distances	Weight	
		Aquatic therapy: UWTM walking 15–30 min SID-BID	Sit-to-stand exercises 10–20 reps BID		
		Swimming 2–5 d per week	Light jogging 3–5 min/d		
		Modalities	Stairs: 2–4 flights SID-BID		
		Heat therapy PRN before activity	Modalities		
		Cryotherapy PRN after exercises	Heat therapy PRN before activity		
			Cryotherapy PRN after exercises		

(continued on next page)

(continued)

Phase	Expected Timeframe[a]	Rehabilitation Clinic Program	Home Program	Outcome Assessment Measures	Criteria for Movement to Next Phase
Trotting at speed with minimal to no lameness	Nine wk postoperative and beyond	Aquatic therapy as desired; otherwise exercises may be continued as part of a home exercise program	Therapeutic exercises pROM for operated limb PRN Leash walks at times and distances tolerated, including fast walks up inclined surfaces Sit-to-stand exercises 20–30 reps as needed Jogging: working up from 10-15 min per day Stairs: walking and trotting, increasing number of flights as tolerated Swimming or walking in mid-to-upper-thigh-level water Ball playing with gradually increasing times and distances, becoming more vigorous over time	Goniometry every 3–4 wk if needed Reevaluate thigh muscle girth every 3–4 wk PRN Response to activity and subjective pain level Lameness score at a stance, walk and trot Weight	Consistent weight bearing on operated limb at a trot; permanent mild gait deficits may persist Minimal to no pain with extensive activities

Abbreviations: PRN, as needed; pROM, passive range of motion; QID, 4 times a day; reps, repetitions; S/S, signs/symptoms; SID, 1 time a day; TID, 3 times a day; UWTM, underwater treadmill.

[a] This protocol is for use by licensed veterinary professionals. It is intended as a guideline, and may be influenced by many factors affecting individualized patient care.

Juvenile Pubic Symphysiodesis

Kathleen A. Linn, DVM, MS

KEYWORDS

- Juvenile pubic symphysiodesis • Hip dysplasia • Hip laxity

KEY POINTS

- In young dogs with lax hips, degenerative joint disease resulting from hip dysplasia may be prevented if hip congruity can be improved and laxity decreased.
- Juvenile pubic symphysiodesis improves hip congruity by producing progressive ventral acetabular rotation and thus better dorsal coverage of the femoral heads. It also reduces hip laxity over time and can halt progression of mild radiographic degenerative changes.
- Juvenile pubic symphysiodesis produces minimal morbidity and causes changes in both hips.
- To be effective, juvenile pubic symphysiodesis must be done in dogs between 12 and 18 weeks of age (slightly older in giant breed dogs) who have mild or moderate hip laxity (ideally, distraction index [DI] ≤ 0.6).

INTRODUCTION

Hip dysplasia is considered a developmental disease: affected puppies are born with apparently normal hips, but laxity of the supporting soft tissues leads to progressive hip subluxation and incongruity, and this incongruity affects the modeling of the acetabula and femoral heads.[1] The resultant increase in slope of the acetabular rims favors dorsolateral movement of the femoral heads during weight bearing, leading to worsening of hip laxity.[2] Interventions that improve dorsal contact between the femoral head and the acetabulum while these bones are growing may forestall the development of degenerative changes. Triple and double pelvic osteotomy techniques do this by rotating the acetabulum ventrally to maximize dorsal coverage of the femoral head.[3,4] Reported success rates for pelvic osteotomy are high if candidates are carefully selected,[4–7] but multiple osteotomies are invasive, require several months of activity restriction after surgery, and have several potential complications.[1,4] In addition, because degenerative changes begin to be evident in dysplastic hips as early as 12 weeks of age,[8] pelvic osteotomies—which are usually done in dogs

Department of Small Animal Clinical Sciences, Western College of Veterinary Medicine, University of Saskatchewan, 52 Campus Drive, Saskatoon, Saskatchewan S7N 5B4, Canada
E-mail address: kathleen.linn@usask.ca

Vet Clin Small Anim 47 (2017) 851–863
http://dx.doi.org/10.1016/j.cvsm.2017.03.004
0195-5616/17/© 2017 Elsevier Inc. All rights reserved.

from 4.5 months to more than a year of age—may come too late to prevent development of osteoarthritis.[1,4–7]

Juvenile pubic symphysiodesis (JPS) is a minimally invasive procedure performed in puppies between 3 and 5 months of age to produce progressive ventrolateral rotation of the acetabula and thus better dorsal femoral head coverage. It takes advantage of the 3-dimensional anatomy of the acetabulum. During development, the acetabulum is formed by the junction of 4 bones: the ilium craniodorsally, the ischium caudodorsally, the pubis ventromedially, and (between 2 and 8 weeks of age) a small acetabular bone centrally. These bones begin to fuse when dogs are around 12 to 18 weeks of age, with the last ossification occurring at the dorsal junction of the ilium and ischium.[9,10] Each pubic bone has 2 cartilage plates, one in the acetabulum and one at the pubic symphysis, that function like physes. The symphyseal cartilage is responsible for most of the longitudinal growth of the pubis, contributing 2 to 4 times more gain in length than the acetabular physis (at least in rats and pigs).[11] If the pubic symphyseal cartilage is prevented from growing as with the JPS procedure, the shortened pubis places a ventromedial constraint on acetabular growth. As the more dorsally located ilium and ischium continue to grow, the acetabulum rotates so that its opening faces more ventrally and the dorsal acetabular rim is more laterally located, resulting in better dorsal coverage of the femoral heads with less tendency for them to subluxate when bearing weight.[4,11] However, because 82% of pelvic growth is complete by 17 weeks of age, JPS must be performed early to be effective.[8,12]

JPS was first proposed as a treatment for hip dysplasia by Mathews and colleagues,[11] who investigated its effects on acetabular positioning and pelvic conformation in guinea pigs. They found that early closure of the pubic symphyseal cartilages led to shortening of the pubic bones with resultant acetabular ventroversion of between 13° and 29°. A controlled study on normal greyhounds by Swainson and colleagues[13] had similar results: JPS produced acetabular ventroversion and decreased hip laxity (as measured by DI). The first trial of JPS on dysplastic canine hips was done in 2001 by Dueland's group[14]; they went on to refine the electrocautery dosage needed for reliable symphysis closure[15] and to investigate optimal timing for JPS.[16]

EFFECTS OF JUVENILE PUBIC SYMPHYSIODESIS

The aim of JPS is to increase acetabular ventroversion, with the expectation that this will decrease the tendency of dysplastic hips to subluxate. If this can be accomplished, hip pain and degenerative changes should be minimized.

Acetabular Ventroversion

Direct measures of acetabular ventroversion include the dorsal acetabular rim angle (DARA), which can be taken from plain radiographs[2,17,18] or transverse computerized tomography (CT) images,[13,14,16] and the acetabular angle (AA), which is taken from transverse CT images at the midpoint of the acetabulum (**Fig. 1**).[12,14,16] Of the 2 CT measures, DARA appears to be less affected by slight differences in patient positioning or slice selection and may thus be the more reliable measure for comparison between different studies.[19]

In all the controlled studies that evaluated changes in acetabular ventroversion after JPS in dysplastic dogs, DARA was significantly reduced (an improvement) at the time of follow-up (by 4°–5° at 6 months after surgery,[20] 6.1° at 1 year, and 7.7° at 2 years after surgery),[12] whereas no changes were seen in unoperated controls. Similarly, AA was significantly improved (by 16° at 1 year of age and by 19° at 2 years of age)

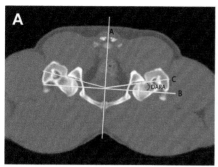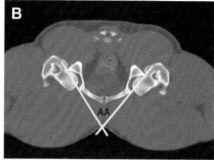

Fig. 1. CT measurements of acetabular ventroversion. (*A*) Measurement of the DARA on a transverse CT image taken at the midpoint of the acetabulum. The yellow lines are drawn across the lateral and medial points of the dorsal acetabular rims. A vertical reference line is drawn through the center of the vertebra to the center of the pelvic symphysis, and a perpendicular horizontal reference line is drawn at the point at which the DARA lines intersect. The DARA for each hip is the angle between this horizontal line and the line across the dorsal acetabular rim. Smaller DARAs indicate increased dorsal acetabular ventroversion. (*B*) Measurement of the AA on a transverse CT image taken at the midpoint of the acetabulum. Lines are drawn from the dorsal acetabular rim to the ventral acetabular rim of each hip and extended ventrally. The AA is the angle made by these lines where they intersect. Larger AAs indicate increased acetabular ventroversion.

in JPS-treated dogs but not in controls (**Fig. 2**).[12] The degree of acetabular ventroversion achieved by JPS was strongly associated with the age at which symphysiodesis was done.[12,14,16,21] Dogs who had JPS performed when they were between 12 and 16 weeks of age (median, 15 weeks) had a mean increase in acetabular angle of 23° at 2 years of age, whereas dogs who were between 19 and 24 weeks of age (median, 20 weeks) at the time of surgery had only a 17° improvement. The period for useful intervention may be a bit longer for giant breed dogs, with meaningful improvements in acetabular ventroversion reported when JPS was done at up to 24 weeks.[12,18,21] Adding pectineus myotomy to JPS in older (18–22 weeks old) dogs does not seem to extend this window of opportunity.[21]

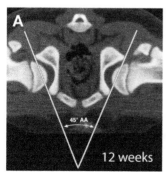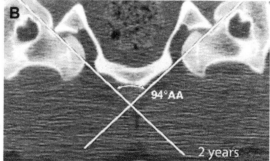

Fig. 2. Acetabular ventroversion produced by JPS. (*A*) AA of a 12-week-old dog just before JPS. (*B*) AA of the same dog at 2 years of age, after JPS surgery. Note the increased AA and the fused pubic symphysis. (*From* Dueland RT, Adams WM, Fialkowski JP, et al. Effects of pubic symphysiodesis in dysplastic puppies. Vet Surg 2001;30(3):201–17; with permission.)

A study comparing long-term effects of JPS with those of triple pelvic osteotomy (TPO)[22] found significant changes in DARA and AA at 2 years of age for TPO but not for JPS. The reason for this difference in results from other studies is unclear, but the inclusion of dogs with relatively severe hip laxity and loss of dogs to follow-up may have played a role.

An experimental study[3] on pelves of young dysplastic dogs that used a hinged TPO plate found that rotating acetabula ventrally by 17.7° to 20° beyond their starting points maximized dorsal coverage of the femoral heads and prevented hip subluxation. The amount of acetabular ventroversion applied in this study was defined by the plate setting rather than being measured via CT. However, because AA represents the combined ventral angulation of both hips, half of the change in AA brought about by JPS should approximate the ventroversion measure from the TPO study. Because dogs receiving JPS at an optimal age experience an average 23° of AA change,[16] ventroversion per hip achieved by JPS seems to be less than the 20° to 25° targeted for pelvic osteotomy techniques.[3,4,22] This does not necessarily mean that JPS is less effective at countering hip subluxation. Because JPS is typically done at a younger age than pelvic osteotomy, it is possible that the earlier intervention is more effective at preventing progression of soft tissue laxity and hip remodeling that contribute to subluxation and therefore requires less ventroversion.

Pelvic Canal Dimensions

In the study on pubic symphysiodesis in guinea pigs, shortening the pubic bones narrowed the pelvic inlet in addition to producing acetabular ventroversion.[11] This also proved to be the case in normal greyhounds, who experienced a decrease in mean pelvic inlet area of 13% relative to control dogs at 11 months of age,[13] and in dysplastic dogs, whose mean pelvic inlet areas were 24% smaller 137 weeks after JPS than those of controls.[14] The narrowed pelvic canal diameter could increase the risk for dystocia in female dogs, one of the reasons sterilization of JPS recipients is recommended. No reports of dystocia or obstipation secondary to JPS have been published, however.

Hip Laxity and Subluxation

- Norberg angle (NA), which is usually measured on ventrodorsal extended-hip views, is a commonly used radiographic index of hip subluxation. NA is the angle formed between a line drawn through the center points of both femoral heads and a line between the femoral head center point and the lateral limit of the dorsal acetabular rim for each hip. An NA less than 105° indicates subluxation of that hip.[23] With one exception,[16] most studies found that JPS led to an increase in NA (usually to normal ranges) over time and compared with final NA in controls.[13,14,16,24]
- DI, measured on stress radiographic views, is a widely accepted measure of hip laxity that predicts the likelihood of a hip developing degenerative joint disease.[25] All studies but one[22] found a decrease in DI after JPS (at least when it is performed before 20 weeks of age).[12–14,16,20,22,24] Another study using a related measure, the Fluckiger subluxation index,[26] found that 85% of dysplastic hips experienced a decrease of the subluxation index to below the dysplastic threshold of 0.5 if JPS was done before 18 weeks of age.[21] It must be noted, however, that in controlled studies, dogs who did not receive JPS also experienced a decrease in DI over time, although to a lesser degree than that of JPS-treated dogs.[12–14] DI is useful in identifying dogs that will best benefit from JPS. In several large case series, Vezzoni and colleagues[18,20] found that

JPS was most effective at restoring normal joint congruity in puppies with a preoperative DI of 0.4 to 0.6 (and best when the DI was <0.5); when DI was greater than 0.6, 55.3% of puppies went on to have moderate or severe degenerative changes (as opposed to 30.9% of puppies with lower initial DI). Dueland and colleagues[27] similarly found that degenerative changes were most likely to progress after JPS in hips with initial DI greater than 0.7. A problem with using this index for JPS case selection, however, is that DI is predictive of the development of degenerative joint disease only after dogs have reached 4 months of age,[25,28,29] and JPS is most effective when done as early as 12 weeks of age.

- Ortolani sign is a physical test for hip laxity that correlates roughly with DI.[2,29,30] The age at which Ortolani sign becomes predictive of persistent hip laxity and degenerative joint disease is unknown. Ortolani sign disappears in at least half of dysplastic dogs after JPS, whereas a smaller proportion of conservatively treated dysplastic dogs have resolution of the positive test.[14,16,22,24] Angle of reduction (AR) and angle of subluxation can be measured during Ortolani testing and may be helpful in identifying dogs who will benefit from JPS[18]; one comparison of various physical and radiographic measures of hip dysplasia found that AR evaluated at 6 months of age was the best predictor of degenerative joint disease at 2 years of age.[2] Most studies following trends in AR over time found a significant decrease in AR (from a preoperative mean angle of 32°–34° to a 2-year mean of 4°–6°) in hips treated with JPS, whereas control hips did not have a significant change in AR.[14,16,27] Interpretation of AR trends over time is difficult, however, as many hips become Ortolani negative, making AR measurement impossible.

Radiographic Evidence of Osteoarthritis

Degenerative joint disease (DJD) is most often evaluated on extended-hip views taken with dogs in dorsal recumbency. Grading scales used for quantification of DJD vary among studies, but all have found lower mean scores at follow-up for hips treated with JPS than for conservatively treated hips and a higher incidence of regression of early degenerative changes (mostly curvilinear osteophytes) in JPS hips.[14,16,18,22,24,27,31] In the largest study, for example, at 12 to 18 months of age, 43.2% of JPS dogs had either regression of degenerative changes or stable radiographic signs, whereas only 23.6% of conservatively treated dogs fell into this category; in contrast, 55.3% of conservatively treated dogs had moderate or severe DJD compared with 30.9% of JPS dogs.[18] The likelihood of development or progression of DJD after JPS was closely associated with the age at which JPS was done (dogs operated on at or before 18 weeks of age fared much better)[18,31] and the degree of hip laxity present at the time of surgery (dogs with initial DI <0.7 had better results, and almost all dogs with DI <0.5 had minimal or no DJD at follow-up).[16,18,27]

Clinical Measures of Hip Pain and Lameness

Lack of radiographic progression of DJD at 1 to 2 years of age has so far been the main experimental criterion for success of JPS and other surgical interventions. However, the real goal of treatment for hip dysplasia is normal, pain-free function—and radiographic changes correlate poorly with clinical signs.[32–34] The effect of an intervention designed to preempt development of hip pain is difficult to test objectively, especially because gait analysis by force plate or pressure platform is difficult to do consistently in little puppies, and results cannot be directly compared between juvenile and adult dogs.[27]

- Pain on hip extension is one clinical sign associated with hip dysplasia that has been tracked in studies evaluating effectiveness of JPS. It is only variably present in the puppies considered the best candidates for the procedure. For example, 85% of dogs treated with JPS in one study did not have evidence of hip pain on preoperative evaluation.[14,21] In another study, 23% of JPS dogs had painful hips before surgery; at the 2-year follow-up evaluation, 6 of 50 JPS hips tested positive for pain. None of the control dogs in this study showed hip pain initially, but 4 of 12 hips in this group were positive for pain at the 2-year point.[27] A series of 10 dogs treated with JPS reported hip pain in all dogs before surgery, but this had resolved in every case by 6 months after surgery.[24]
- Owner questionnaires and subjective lameness examinations have been used in 2 studies to track activity and function in JPS dogs. In a study comparing the effects of TPO with those of JPS, all dogs in both groups had slight to marked difficulties getting around before surgery, according to their owners. At the time of the 2-year follow-up, most dogs in both groups were rated as having only slight difficulties. The dogs treated with TPO significantly improved in lameness scores over preoperative values. This effect was not seen with JPS dogs, but at the 2-year follow-up there was no difference between the groups in overall lameness scores.[22] Another study found that 85% of owner questionnaire/activity score results "normalized" (in combination with other parameters) for dogs receiving JPS before 17 weeks of age, whereas only 15% to 27% of control dogs and dogs receiving JPS after 17 weeks of age had normalized scores at 3 to 4 months of age.[21]
- To date, the only objective assessment of gait after JPS has been by force plate testing done at 1 or 2 years of age. Studies comparing JPS and control dogs have shown normal results for both groups.[14,16] There was no difference in peak vertical force between dogs treated with JPS and dogs treated with TPO, but TPO dogs did have a significantly lower vertical impulse than did JPS dogs 2 years after surgery.[22]

CASE SELECTION

JPS surgery should be performed in dogs that are between 12 and 18 weeks of age.[12,14,18,21,31] This period of opportunity may extend to approximately 22 weeks of age in giant breed dogs, who grow more slowly and for a longer period.[18,21] As JPS is relatively ineffective in correcting severe hip laxity, DI should be less than 0.75 and ideally within the range of 0.4 to 0.6.[12,18] Puppies with distraction indices greater than 0.6 should be operated on as close to 12 weeks of age as possible.[12] No single parameter is completely predictive of postoperative DJD, so it is recommended to use several in deciding whether JPS is an appropriate treatment; for best results, candidates should have positive Ortolani sign with AR between 15° and 35°, angle of subluxation between 0° and 10°, and DARA between 7° and 10°.[18]

A problem with this strategy is that many puppies fitting these criteria show no clinical signs. Dogs that would benefit from JPS may not be presented for treatment until it is too late. Distraction index is only reliably predictive of DJD development when it exceeds 0.7,[28] and even so, most dogs with radiographic evidence of hip DJD are judged by their owners to have normal mobility[32–34]; therefore, JPS should be considered more a preemptive intervention than a therapeutic one. A useful approach might be to screen puppies at 12 weeks of age; for those with positive Ortolani sign or close relatives known to have hip dysplasia, further testing and potential surgery can be recommended.[12]

SURGICAL TECHNIQUE
Approach

A ventral midline or parapreputial incision is made starting at the palpable cranial aspect of the pubis and extending caudally 3 to 5 cm. Sharp dissection is used to divide subcutaneous and fascial tissue on midline until the pubic symphysis is reached. Soft tissues (adductor muscles) can be elevated a few millimeters to either side using a periosteal elevator or a scalpel. The cartilage of the symphysis is usually apparent as a line that is slightly darker than the surrounding bone, and a 25-gauge hypodermic needle can be easily passed into it. The symphysis is exposed along the bases of the pubic rami; a useful caudal landmark is a small, palpable tubercle on the medial edge of both obturator foramina that marks the end of the pubic symphysis and the beginning of the ischial symphysis. The area of cartilage destruction will stretch from the cranial edge of the pubic symphysis to the level of these small tubercles (**Fig. 3**), a distance of about 1.5 cm in most dogs.[12]

Ablation of the Symphysis

There are many ways to bring about pubic symphysiodesis. Resection of the cartilage of the symphysis, or resection combined with stapling across the pubis, arrests symphyseal growth.[11,13] Stapling across the symphysis without resection, however, does not appear to be effective.[13] Most JPS techniques use electrosurgery or radiofrequency ablation to cause thermal necrosis of the symphyseal cartilage.

Bipolar electrosurgery applied in a transverse fashion across the symphysis causes cartilage necrosis in guinea pigs,[11] but because it may not be effective across larger symphyses, monopolar electrocautery is generally used in dogs. Electrosurgery can be applied to the symphyseal cartilage in coagulation mode with a spatula-tip electrode at 30 W in multiple 5- to 10-second bursts,[12,14] although it creates a charred area that can be up to a centimeter in width (**Fig. 4**). Radiofrequency ablation (applied with a spatula electrode in coagulation mode at 50 W in 7–8 second bursts) is also effective.[18]

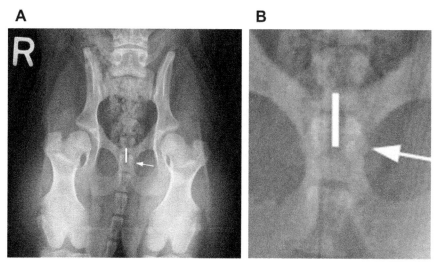

A   **B**

Fig. 3. Landmarks for JPS. (*A*) The white arrow shows the small tubercle along the medial aspect of the obturator foramen that marks the caudal extent of the pubis. The white line shows the area of symphysis to be ablated. (*B*) A close up view shows the small tubercle in detail.

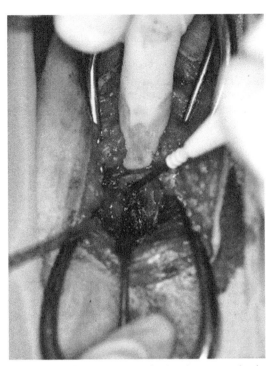

Fig. 4. Electrosurgery ablation of the pubic symphysis using a spatula electrode. Cranial is to the top of the picture. Note the finger placed through a small incision to protect structures dorsal to the pubis. (*Courtesy of* Tass Dueland, DVM, MS, DACVS, Pres ACVS, University of Wisconsin School of Veterinary, Madison, WI.)

Application of electrosurgery via a needle electrode placed through the cartilage in multiple sites generally causes less char than does spatula electrosurgery (**Fig. 5**). The needle electrode is placed at 2- to 3-mm intervals along the midline through the width of the symphyseal cartilage, avoiding penetration of the needle's tip through the periosteum on the dorsal surface of the pubis. 40 W applied for 12 to 20 seconds at each location is generally enough to cause full-thickness cartilage necrosis.[12,15] Depth of needle placement is confirmed with a finger introduced via transrectal palpation[16,18,20] or through an incision in the linea alba or prepubic tendon just cranial to the pubis.[18,21] Saline lavage is used after each cautery application to cool the tissues surrounding the symphysis.[16,18,20] Nevertheless, it gets very hot dorsal to the pubis, so it is important to protect the urethra and rectum during current application. If an incision has been made cranial to the pubis, either the surgeon's finger or a nonconductive object like a wooden spatula is interposed between the dorsal aspect of the pubis and the structures within the pelvic canal.[18] If transrectal palpation is used, the finger within the rectum is used to move the urethra and the rectum off to the side.[12,15,21]

If the prepubic tendon or linea alba has been incised, it is closed with a few interrupted sutures. Closure of the approach incision is routine.

Aftercare

Analgesics are given perioperatively and for a few days after surgery. Some investigators recommend that dogs be kept in a confined area and their exercise limited to walks on a leash for 2 weeks to 2 months after surgery.[12,18,20,21] Others, however,

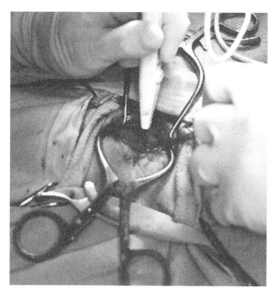

Fig. 5. Electrosurgery ablation of the pubic symphysis using a needle electrode. Cranial is to the top of the picture. The right hand of the surgeon holding the cautery handle has been placed under the drape and into the rectum to confirm needle placement and then move the rectum and urethra out of the way while current is being applied. (*Courtesy of* Tass Duel-and, DVM, MS, DACVS, Pres ACVS, University of Wisconsin School of Veterinary, Madison, WI.)

impose no exercise restrictions.[15,16] Results and complication rates are similar in both cases.

COMPLICATIONS

Complications of JPS are rare[13,14,20,24] and most are quite minor. Postoperative lameness is not to be expected. Seroma formation or mild pain at the incision site is occasionally noted,[21] and when transrectal palpation has been used to confirm needle electrode placement, puppies often have loose or mucoid stools for a day after surgery.[12,16] No injuries to the urethra or rectum have been reported.

Burns at the site of the monopolar electrosurgery grounding plate have been reported in 6 dogs.[12,18,35] These were all associated with poor contact between part of the grounding plate and the skin. To avoid this complication, hair should be clipped and vacuumed away from the site before the grounding plate is applied, and use of adhesive gel plates should be considered; care should be taken to ensure that the grounding plate size is appropriate for the patient. Alternatively, radiofrequency ablation could be used instead of electrosurgery, as no burns have been reported with this modality.[18]

RADIOGRAPHIC CHARACTERISTICS OF JUVENILE PUBIC SYMPHYSIODESIS PELVES

Mandatory sterilization of all dogs receiving JPS is recommended[18,35] for several reasons. First, the narrowed pelvic inlet diameter associated with JPS has the potential to impede normal delivery of puppies in female dogs. Of more concern, however, is the heritable nature of canine hip dysplasia. Because JPS does not use implants that are visible on radiographs, this procedure might make it easier for genotypically dysplastic (but clinically normal) dogs to enter breeding programs undetected.[21]

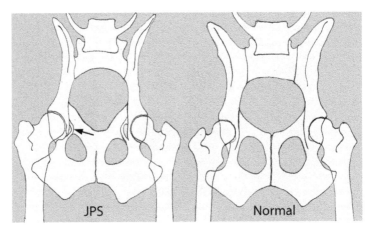

Fig. 6. Radiographic differences between JPS and normal pelves after 1 year of age. The JPS pelvis is depicted on the left and a normal pelvis is on the right. Note the loss of the pubic symphysis line, the thickened and irregular pubic rami, the relatively circular obturator foramina, and the pronounced medial projection of the acetabular fossa (*arrow*) in the JPS pelvis.

Because JPS is a short procedure, concurrent gonadectomy is easy enough to do. However, several large surveys have found a higher incidence of hip dysplasia in dogs that have been spayed or castrated.[36–38] This effect seems to be most marked in males neutered before 5.5 months of age.[39] Given these findings, concurrent gonadectomy has the potential to work against what JPS is trying to accomplish.

Although JPS does not leave implants to document that the procedure has been done, there are subtle changes to the pelvis that occur after this operation[40] that serve as reliable markers (**Fig. 6**). The most easily detected changes include:

- Loss of lucency in the pubic portion of the symphysis; in normal dogs symphyseal lucency is present for at least 2 years.[10]
- Shortening and thickening of the pubic rami. These are also often irregular and asymmetric in dogs that have had JPS.
- The medial projection of the acetabular fossae becomes more prominent owing to acetabular ventroversion.
- The obturator foramina become wider (more circular) relative to their normal oval shape.

SUMMARY

In properly selected dogs, JPS improves joint congruity, decreases hip laxity, and can reverse or prevent progression of degenerative joint disease in the hips. Advantages it holds over other surgical treatments for hip dysplasia are its minimal morbidity (and expense), ability to treat both hips with one intervention, and ability to prevent secondary effects of hip dysplasia from occurring. However, to be effective, it must be done at a very young age (12–18 weeks) and in hips that are only mildly to moderately lax. Because many dogs that might benefit from JPS are asymptomatic during the appropriate window of time, JPS is perhaps best viewed more as a preemptive procedure than as a strictly therapeutic one. Dogs considered to be at risk for hip dysplasia should be screened with Ortolani testing at 12 weeks of age, with further imaging and perhaps surgery to follow for those who have a positive Ortolani sign.

REFERENCES

1. Piermattei DL, Flo GL, DeCamp CE. Brinker, Piermattei and Flo's handbook of small animal orthopedics and fracture repair. 4th edition. St Louis (MO): Saunders Elsevier; 2006.
2. Gatineau M, Dupuis J, Beauregard G, et al. Palpation and dorsal rim radiographic projection for early detection of canine hip dysplasia: a prospective study. Vet Surg 2012;41(1):42–53.
3. Dejardin LM, Perry RL, Arnoczky SP. The effect of triple pelvic osteotomy on the articular contact area of the hip joint in dysplastic dogs: an *in vitro* experimental study. Vet Surg 1998;27(3):194–202.
4. Vezzoni A, Boiocchi S, Vezzoni L, et al. Double pelvic osteotomy for the treatment of hip dysplasia in young dogs. Vet Comp Orthop Traumatol 2010;23(6):444–52.
5. Slocum B, Devine T. Pelvic osteotomy in the dog as treatment for hip dysplasia. Semin Vet Med Surg 1987;2:107–16.
6. McLaughlin RM, Miller CW, Taves CL, et al. Force plate analysis of triple pelvic osteotomy for the treatment of canine hip dysplasia. Vet Surg 1991;20(5):291–7.
7. Rasmussen LM, Kramek BA, Lipowitz AJ. Preoperative variables affecting long-term outcome of triple pelvic osteotomy for treatment of naturally occurring hip dysplasia in dogs. J Am Vet Med Assoc 1998;213(1):80–5.
8. Riser WH. Growth and development of the normal canine pelvis, hip joints and femurs from birth to maturity. Vet Path 1975;12:264–78.
9. Evans HE, deLahunta A. Miller's anatomy of the dog. 4th edition. St Louis (MO): Saunders Elsevier; 2013.
10. Smith RN. The pelvis of the young dog. Vet Rec 1964;76(6):975–9.
11. Mathews KG, Stover SM, Kass PH. Effect of pubic symphysiodesis on acetabular rotation and pelvic development in guinea pigs. Am J Vet Res 1996;57(10): 1427–33.
12. Dueland RT, Adams WM, Patricelli AJ, et al. Canine hip dysplasia treated by juvenile pubic symphysiodesis. Part 1: two year results of computed tomography and distraction index. Vet Comp Orthop Traumatol 2010;23:306–17.
13. Swainson SS, Conzemius MG, Riedesel EA, et al. Effect of pubic symphysiodesis on pelvic development in the skeletally immature greyhound. Vet Surg 2000; 29(2):178–90.
14. Dueland RT, Adams WM, Fialkowski JP, et al. Effects of pubic symphysiodesis in dysplastic puppies. Vet Surg 2001;30(3):201–17.
15. Patricelli AJ, Dueland RT, Lu Y, et al. Canine pubic symphysiodesis: investigation of electrocautery dose response by histologic examination and temperature measurement. Vet Surg 2001;30(3):261–8.
16. Patricelli AJ, Dueland RT, Adams WM, et al. Juvenile pubic symphysiodesis in dysplastic puppies at 15 and 20 weeks of age. Vet Surg 2002;31(5):435–44.
17. Slocum B, Devine TM. Dorsal acetabular rim radiographic view for evaluation of the canine hip. J Am Anim Hosp Assoc 1990;26:289–96.
18. Vezzoni A, Dravelli G, Vezzoni L, et al. Comparison of conservative management and juvenile pubic symphysiodesis in the early treatment of canine hip dysplasia. Vet Comp Orthop Traumatol 2008;21(3):267–79.
19. Wang SI, Mathews KG, Robertson LD, et al. The effects of patient positioning and slice selection on canine acetabular angle assessment with computerized tomography. Vet Radiol Ultrasound 2005;46(1):39–43.

20. Vezzoni A, Magni G, De Lorenzi M, et al. Pubic symphysiodesis: clinical experiences. In Proc 1st World Orthop Vet Congress ESVOT-VOS, Munich 2002, 204–207.
21. Bernardé A. Juvenile pubic symphysiodesis and juvenile pubic symphysiodesis with pectineus myotomy: short-term outcome in 56 dysplastic puppies. Vet Surg 2010;39:158–64.
22. Manley PM, Adams WM, Danielson KC, et al. Long-term outcome of juvenile pubic symphysiodesis and triple pelvic osteotomy in dogs with hip dysplasia. J Am Vet Med Assoc 2007;230(2):206–10.
23. Culp WT, Kapatkin AS, Gregor TP, et al. Evaluation of the Norberg angle threshold: a comparison of Norberg angle and distraction index as measures of coxofemoral degenerative joint disease susceptibility in seven breeds of dogs. Vet Surg 2006;35(5):453–9.
24. Özdemir G, Bilgili H. Alterations in hip angles following of juvenile pubic symphysiodesis in ten dogs with hip dysplasia. Kafkas Univ Vet Fak Derg 2011;17(3): 393–400.
25. Smith GK, Gregor TP, Rhodes WH, et al. Coxofemoral joint laxity from distraction radiography and its contemporaneous and prospective correlation with laxity, subjective score, and evidence of degenerative joint disease from conventional hip-extended radiography in dogs. Am J Vet Res 1993;54:1021–42.
26. Fluckiger MA, Friedrich GA, Binder H. A radiographic stress test for evaluation of coxofemoral joint laxity in dogs. Vet Surg 1999;28(1):1–9.
27. Dueland RT, Patricelli AJ, Adams WM, et al. Canine hip dysplasia treated by juvenile pubic symphysiodesis. Part II: two year clinical results. Vet Comp Orthop Traumatol 2010;23:318–25.
28. Smith GK, Popovitch CA, Gregor TP, et al. Evaluation of risk factors for degenerative joint disease associated with hip dysplasia in dogs. J Am Vet Med Assoc 1996;91:26–33.
29. Adams WM, Dueland RT, Daniels R, et al. Comparison of two palpation, four radiographic and three ultrasound methods for early detection of mild to moderate hip dysplasia. Vet Radiol Ultrasound 2000;41:484–90.
30. Adama WM, Dueland RT, Meinen J, et al. Early detection of canine hip dysplasia: comparison of two palpation and five radiographic methods. J Am Anim Hosp Assoc 1998;34:339–47.
31. Vezzoni A, Dravelli G, Delorenzi M, et al. Efficacia della sinfisiodesi pubica giovanile (JPS) nel trattamento precoce della dysplasia nel cane. Efficacy of juvenile pubic symphysiodesis in the early treatment of canine hip dysplasia. Veterinaria 2006;20(6):9–28.
32. Fry TR, Clark DM. Canine hip dysplasia: clinical signs and diagnosis. Vet Clin North Am Small Anim Pract 1992;22:551–8.
33. Tomlinson J, McLaughlin R. Canine hip dysplasia: developmental factors, clinical signs, and initial examination steps. Vet Med 1996;91:26–33.
34. Tomlinson J, McLaughlin R. Medically managing canine hip dysplasia. Vet Med 1996;91:48–53.
35. Mathews KG. Juvenile pubic symphysiodesis—what we do and don't know. Proc North Am Vet Conf 2006;932–3.
36. Torres de la Riva G, Hart BL, Farver TB, et al. Neutering dogs: effects on joint disorders and cancers in golden retrievers. PLoS One 2013;8(2):e55937.
37. Duerr FM, Duncan CG, Savicky RS, et al. Risk factors for excessive tibial plateau angle in large-breed dogs with cranial cruciate ligament disease. J Am Vet Med Assoc 2007;231(11):1688–91.

38. van Hagen MA, Ducro BJ, van den Broek J, et al. Incidence, risk factors, and heritability estimates of hind limb lameness caused by hip dysplasia in a birth cohort of boxers. Am J Vet Res 2005;66(2):307–12.
39. Spain CV, Scarlett JM, Houpt KA. Long-term risks and benefits of early-age gonadectomy in dogs. J Am Vet Med Assoc 2004;224(3):380–7.
40. Boiocchi S, Vezzoni L, Vezzoni A, et al. Radiographic changes of the pelvis in Labrador and golden retrievers after juvenile pubic symphysiodesis. Vet Comp Orthop Traumatol 2013;26:218–25.

Triple Pelvic Osteotomy and Double Pelvic Osteotomy

Francisco Guevara, DVM, Samuel P. Franklin, MS, DVM, PhD*

KEYWORDS

- TPO • Triple pelvic osteotomy • DPO • Double pelvic osteotomy • Hip dysplasia
- Dog

KEY POINTS

- Corrective osteotomies of the pelvis have been used for decades as an early intervention for dysplastic hips in young canine patients.
- Multiple variations of the procedure are in clinical use, and the two most commonly used are the triple pelvic osteotomy (TPO) and the double pelvic osteotomy (DPO).
- Both the TPO and DPO are designed to improve acetabular ventro-version and femoral head coverage.
- Improvements in technique and implants over the last several years seem to have resulted in decreasing prevalence of complications.
- The data suggest that pelvic osteotomies commonly improve clinical function but that osteoarthritis is typically progressive.

Canine hip dysplasia (CHD) is a complex orthopedic condition characterized by hip laxity with concurrent or consequent maldevelopment of the osseous joint structures. These abnormalities often result in varying degrees of joint instability, femoral head subluxation, pain, lameness, and osteoarthritis (OA). Pelvic osteotomies are elective orthopedic procedures designed to increase acetabular ventro-version and minimize femoral head subluxation in dogs with excess hip laxity. In addition to increased dorsal acetabular coverage, immediate technical aims of pelvic osteotomy techniques may include improved congruency between the central acetabulum and femoral head and more favorable loading of the articular cartilage. These concepts were originally introduced in the early 1960s for the treatment of children with congenital dislocations of the hip,[1–3] and Hohn and Janes[4] described the first veterinary application of pelvic

Disclosure Statement: The authors have nothing to disclose.
Department of Small Animal Medicine and Surgery, University of Georgia College of Veterinary Medicine, 2200 College Station Road, Athens, GA 30602, USA
* Corresponding author.
E-mail address: spfrank@uga.edu

osteotomies for the treatment of CHD in 1969. The initial surgical techniques have been modified over the ensuing decades, but all current pelvic osteotomy techniques retain the same mechanical goal of increasing dorsal acetabular coverage of the femoral head via axial rotation of the acetabular segment.

PROCEDURE CLINICAL OBJECTIVES

Although all variations of the pelvic osteotomy procedure share the same mechanical objectives, there are disparate clinical objectives that are surgeon dependent and in turn affect both patient selection and whether one considers these surgeries to be commonly successful or not. During the time of its introduction to veterinary surgery, the objectives described for triple pelvic osteotomy (TPO) were to increase dorsal acetabular coverage of the femoral head, provide stability, and to provide pain relief and restoration of function to dysplastic canine patients.[5] Furthermore, pelvic osteotomy was suggested as potentially preventing the onset or progression of OA, particularly when performed in young patients before the initiation of OA.[5] The goals of eliminating any subluxation and preventing OA are lofty objectives and certainly not obtainable in all patients. Conversely, more recent studies have focused on mitigating, rather than eliminating, subluxation and improving function rather than completely preventing inception or progression of OA.[6] These points are important to consider, as the desired goals influence patient selection and categorizations of successful or unsuccessful outcomes.

Evaluation and Selection of Surgical Candidates

Numerous patient characteristics are often considered in selecting candidates for pelvic osteotomy. The most frequently considered criteria are the severity of lameness, signalment, osseous conformation, degree of hip laxity, and the severity of secondary changes already present, including damage to the acetabular labrum, ligament of the head of the femur, and articular cartilage. In addition, the desired goals of the procedure must be considered in conjunction with patients' characteristics to determine how likely pelvic osteotomy is to achieve a successful result in each individual.

LAMENESS

A relevant question is whether pelvic osteotomy should be performed exclusively in dogs with clinical signs of pain and lameness or whether it is appropriate to include dogs without clinical signs of lameness but with suboptimal hip laxity. Some surgeons do not recommend performing pelvic osteotomy on dogs without current clinical signs, citing uncertainty as to whether such dogs will ever develop clinical signs associated with hip dysplasia or the severity of such clinical signs if they arise. Conversely, some surgeons perform pelvic osteotomies on dogs with excess hip laxity with the goals of preventing the onset of lameness and/or preventing secondary OA and osseous remodeling. The rationale for the latter approach is based in part on the fact that there is no cure for OA. Therefore, prevention of lameness and OA, at least theoretically, is preferable to clinical management of lameness and OA after they are present. This vantage point is particularly appealing if one thinks that treatment with pelvic osteotomy is superior to the treatments available for dogs with hip OA, which are currently limited to nonsurgical management, femoral head and neck excision (FHNE), or total hip replacement (THR). However, the uncertainty that lameness or OA will ever occur, along with the likelihood that pelvic osteotomy could prevent lameness and/or OA development, and the associated costs and risk associated with the surgery should all be considered when deciding whether pelvic osteotomy should be performed on sound patients.

Although owners' and veterinarians' subjective assessment of lameness are important components of patient selection for pelvic osteotomies, it is also relevant to discuss the limitations of such selection methodology. Multiple studies have demonstrated that owners and veterinarians are relatively inconsistent and inaccurate when assessing lameness subjectively in comparison with objective measures of function using force plates, particularly when lameness is subtle.[7–9] Therefore, it is feasible that some dogs that are considered sound by owners and veterinarians on subjective assessment might truly have a degree of lameness or dysfunction that is just not visually detectable. Objective assessment of gait could theoretically be used to determine whether dogs with excess hip laxity, and for whom pelvic osteotomy is being considered, are truly sound. Force plates are not commonly used in practice and require dedicated space for their placement. Alternatively, portable pressure-sensitive mats are increasingly common and could contribute to patient selection.[10,11] Similarly, objective kinetic data can be used to assess response to treatment.

Finally, the authors are unaware of any suggestion that some dogs may be too lame to be candidates for pelvic osteotomy. However, most dogs that are treated tend to have mild to moderate lameness. The presence of severe or non–weight-bearing lameness should prompt consideration of alternative explanations for the lameness and the applicability of pelvic osteotomy.

SIGNALMENT

Pelvic osteotomy procedures are most commonly performed in juvenile, large to giant breed dogs, although successful outcomes have been reported in smaller breeds of dogs following TPO.[12] Age is commonly cited as a selection criterion, but often this is used as a rough guideline or surrogate for assessing the likelihood that the dog already has secondary OA and osseous conformational abnormalities. The probability and severity of secondary OA increases with age; older dogs are less likely to have suitable osseous conformation and cartilage quality. As a result, pelvic osteotomy procedures are almost exclusively performed in younger dogs ranging from 5 to 14 months of age, with most being younger than 1 year.

HIP LAXITY

The most relevant physical examination finding in regard to pelvic osteotomy procedures is the identification of hip laxity. Hip laxity can rarely be appreciated during gait analysis and is most commonly identified by performing the Ortolani test on sedated or anesthetized patients.[13] A positive Ortolani sign is abnormal and consistent with suboptimal hip laxity. The angle of subluxation (AS) and angle of reduction (AR), which can be measured with a goniometer, have been used to provide an estimate of the quantity of acetabular ventro-version required to adequately increase dorsal coverage of the femoral head. The AS and AR may also correlate with laxity.[5,6] Consequently, high angles of reduction and subluxation can potentially be used to conclude that pelvic osteotomy is unlikely to provide adequate femoral head coverage and successfully prevent femoral head subluxation.[14] However, repeatability of these measurements, their correlations to the amount of ventro-version required, and their correlation with postoperative functional outcomes have not been established to the authors' knowledge. Similarly, the absence of an Ortolani sign is not sufficient to rule out increased hip laxity.[15] Thus, more repeatable and quantifiable methods of assessing hip laxity have been developed.[15]

Distraction radiography, such as the PennHIP method, provides an objective and repeatable assessment of hip laxity by quantifying the distraction index (DI; **Fig. 1**).[16] Studies have shown that increasing degrees of hip laxity, as measured by DI, is correlated with the probability that a dog will develop radiographic OA later in life.[17] DI values have also been used to establish susceptibility curves for several specific dog breeds that are commonly affected by CHD.[18,19] Accordingly, DIs can be used to quantify the degree of hip laxity in a given patient and could theoretically be used as a selection criterion for pelvic osteotomy. However, no studies have established what DIs should be used for patient selection. Furthermore, it is not clear whether an appropriate candidate is a dog with minimal, moderate, or severe hip laxity. An argument against performing pelvic osteotomy in a dog with minimal hip laxity, manifest as a relatively low DI, would include that the dog is unlikely to develop clinical signs associated with OA. Conversely, an argument against treating a dog with severe hip laxity is that pelvic osteotomy may be unlikely in such case to prevent femoral head subluxation as has been documented clinically.[6] In turn, the degree of laxity that a candidate for pelvic osteotomy should have depends to some extent on the perceived objectives of the procedure.

OSSEOUS CONFORMATION

Pelvic radiographs, including pelvic limb extended ventrodorsal (VD), VD with legs abducted (also known as frog leg), lateral pelvis, and dorsal acetabular rim (DAR) views, can all be evaluated and beneficial in assessing anatomic conformation and secondary changes of the coxofemoral joint (**Figs. 1–3**).[20–22] Measures of femoral head coverage by the dorsal acetabulum that can be made from the VD legs

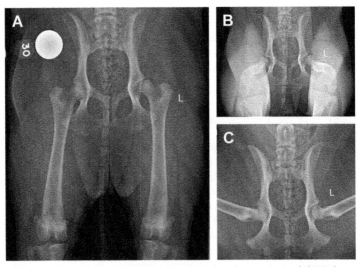

Fig. 1. Patient A: A 10-month-old spayed female Labrador retriever. (*A*) VD legs extended view demonstrating minimal to no femoral head subluxation of the right femoral head (*left in the image*) with mild to moderate femoral head subluxation on the left. (*B*) Distraction radiography technique documenting substantial hip laxity bilaterally. (*C*) VD legs abducted view (also known as frog leg) demonstrating good congruency on the right and reduced congruency on the left.

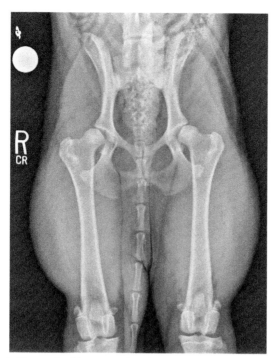

Fig. 2. Patient B: A 10-month-old castrated male golden retriever. VD legs extended view demonstrating moderate femoral head subluxation bilaterally. Note the lack of radiographic evidence of OA. Diagnostic coxofemoral arthroscopy was performed bilaterally and confirmed intact dorsal labrums with no cartilage erosion bilaterally. The dog had intermittent lameness according to the owner.

extended view include the percent of femoral head coverage (PC) and Norberg angle (NA); these also provide some, albeit relatively poor, assessment of hip laxity.[23] Similarly, the radiographic DAR view also provides an assessment of femoral head coverage as do measures of the DAR angles and acetabular angles made on

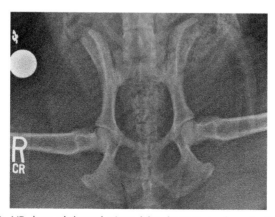

Fig. 3. Patient B: VD legs abducted view (also known as frog leg) demonstrating a subjectively high level of congruency present.

cross-sectional images using computed tomography (CT).[20,21,24,25] Given that an accepted and universal goal of pelvic osteotomy is to improve femoral head coverage, these imaging modalities can be used to identify dogs that have abnormal conformation with minimal femoral head coverage. However, the exact PC, NA, DAR, and acetabular angles that should be used to select surgical candidates have not been established.

The congruency index (CI) is measured on a VD view with the limbs abducted and force applied to direct the femoral heads into the acetabulum (see **Figs. 1C and 3**).[22] This view depicts the ideal seating of the femoral head within the acetabulum and their congruency. Additional assessment of the osseous conformation can be made subjectively by evaluating the shape and depth of the acetabulum and shape of the femoral head. In general, it has been suggested that candidates for pelvic osteotomy should have well-formed osseous structures with high congruency despite inadequate femoral head coverage and excessive laxity. This recommendation corresponds with a desired goal of improving femoral head coverage and decreasing femoral head subluxation. In turn, it seems intuitive that dogs with poor conformation, poor congruency, and substantial subluxation on VD radiographs would be poor candidates for pelvic osteotomy. However, defined criteria for the PC, NA, CI, and DAR have not been established; surgeons must use the information garnered from these diagnostics tests without specific guidelines.

DEGREE OF JOINT DAMAGE

Pelvic osteotomy, as suggested earlier, has been used as a joint-preservation procedure with the goals of preventing femoral head subluxation and the initiation of OA. Achieving such goals requires accurate preoperative identification and exclusion of dogs with irreversible and incipient joint damage, which will progress regardless of whether pelvic osteotomy is performed. In turn, assessment of joint health has received substantial attention as it pertains to patient selection with particular emphasis placed on the integrity of the dorsal acetabular labrum and the articular cartilage.

The dorsal acetabular labrum and cartilage health can potentially be assessed, to a small degree, with physical palpation. The presence of crepitus and a less distinct click on reduction during an Ortolani test have been suggested to correlate with damage to the dorsal labrum.[13] Despite a correlation between degree of degenerative change and physical palpation of laxity, whether one can consistently or accurately characterize health of the labrum on physical examination is uncertain.[15] However, substantial crepitus is consistent with OA and suggests that patients are unlikely to be candidates for pelvic osteotomy and definitively not if prevention of OA is a desired goal of the procedure.

The most common method for assessing the presence or severity of OA is radiography. If any signs of OA are identified radiographically, the progression of OA is likely regardless of whether pelvic osteotomy is performed.[26,27] Unfortunately, radiography is not sensitive for detecting relevant joint damage, both in the hip and shoulder, and so the absence of these radiographic findings does not equate with a healthy joint.[28,29] Fifty percent of canine hips with moderate cartilage damage as assessed arthroscopically were unremarkable radiographically.[28] In addition, assessment of specific radiographic markers of OA is only fairly repeatable even among experienced observers.[30] Therefore, if cartilage health is to be used as a selection criterion for pelvic osteotomy, additional diagnostics are necessary.

One study demonstrated a correlation between histologic assessments of cartilage quality in 12 hips and measurements of anatomic configuration and laxity using CT, suggesting that CT could be superior to radiography in predicting hip damage.[31] However, the gold standard for assessing cartilage health in the hip is arthroscopy; some surgeons recommend that arthroscopy be performed to stage disease.[28,32] Arthroscopic confirmation of healthy cartilage (**Fig. 4**) is likely a critical step in patient selection if preventing onset of OA is an objective. However, if the surgical objectives do not include prevention of OA, arthroscopy may not be considered a necessary part of the patient evaluation.[6] As with the aforementioned staging tools, specific selection criteria, such as the acceptable level of arthroscopic cartilage pathologic change (**Fig. 5**), have not been established.

SUMMARIZED CONSIDERATIONS FOR PATIENT SELECTION

Several patient characteristics can be considered when determining whether patients are good candidates for pelvic osteotomy. Despite the lack of rigid criteria for patient selection, some suggested guidelines are proposed. Dogs with extreme laxity are unlikely to be good candidates because the procedure is unlikely to prevent persistent femoral head subluxation. Similarly, dogs with virtually absent femoral head coverage and a severely damaged dorsal acetabular labrum are likely poor candidates because adequate femoral head coverage is unlikely to be obtained. Furthermore, dogs with substantial OA are suboptimal candidates because the OA will not be resolved with the surgery and the presence of OA may contribute to persistent pain and dysfunction. Whether dogs must be lame to justify the surgery, how one characterizes laxity and how much laxity is ideal, and how degenerative change is characterized and used as a selection tool are all otherwise not established.

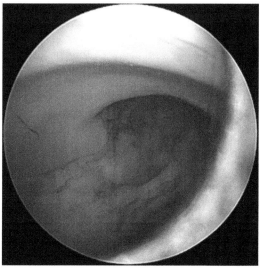

Fig. 4. Patient B: Arthroscopic image of the right coxofemoral joint. The cartilage of the acetabulum and dorsal rim appears unremarkable.

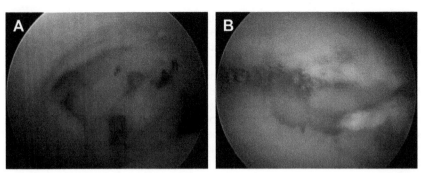

Fig. 5. Patient A: (A) Arthroscopic image of the right coxofemoral joint. The cartilage of the acetabulum and dorsal rim appears unremarkable. This hip was considered appropriate for pelvic osteotomy. (B) Arthroscopic image of the left coxofemoral joint. There is fraying of the labrum and focal full-thickness cartilage loss (Outerbridge grade III damage) on the dorsal rim. This hip was not considered appropriate for pelvic osteotomy.

Surgical Technique

There are 2 variations of the pelvic osteotomy procedure that are currently described and in clinical use. The TPO is the most thoroughly described and the double pelvic osteotomy (DPO) is a recent variation that differs from the more traditional TPO in that the ischium is not cut. There is also a third variation, the 2.5 pelvic osteotomy (2.5 PO), that has been described in a cadaveric study but has not yet been described clinically. Regardless of whether a TPO or DPO is performed, much of the technique is identical.

Approach to the ischium

- Patients are placed in lateral recumbency; a horizontal incision is made directly over the caudal aspect of the ischium, parallel to the ischial table and just medial to the ischiatic tuberosity. Sharp incision is extended onto the caudal aspect of the ischium, and the internal obturator muscle is elevated from the dorsal surface of the ischium. Similarly, the musculature on the ventral aspect of the ischium is elevated until the obturator foramen is reached. Hohmann retractors may be placed, one dorsally and one ventrally, with the tips in the obturator foramen. An osteotomy of the isolated ischial table is then performed with Gigli wire or oscillating saw. The osteotomy ideally extends from approximately the caudo-lateral border of the obturator foramen through the ischiatic table medial to the ischiatic tuberosity (**Fig. 6**). If hemi-cerclage wire is to be used, holes are drilled on either side of the ischial osteotomy and the wire is loosely placed, to be secured after rotation of the acetabular segment is achieved.

Approach to the pubis

- For bilateral simultaneous procedures, patients may be placed in dorsal recumbency otherwise they are usually in lateral recumbency. When in lateral recumbency the pelvic limb is held in abduction by an assistant to allow access to the inguinal region. A skin incision is made parallel to the caudal edge of the pectineus muscle, from approximately its origin on the pelvic symphysis to beyond the coxofemoral joint. Blunt dissection is performed directly caudal and parallel to the pectineus and the pectineus is retracted cranially. The pectineus does not need to be transected or released in order to reach the pubis.[6]

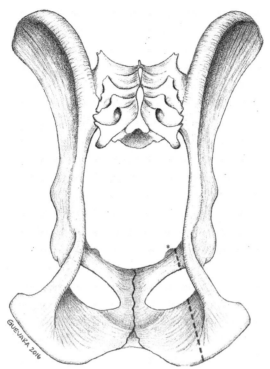

Fig. 6. Canine pelvis (caudo-dorsal view) demonstrating the relative locations of pubic and ischial osteotomies (*dashed lines*). The pubic osteotomy is ideally performed immediately abaxial to the iliopubic eminence (*asterisk*) and immediately axial to the acetabulum. The iliopubic eminence is most prominent on the ventral aspect of the pubis and is identifiable intraoperatively.

- A Hohmann retractor is placed with its tip immediately cranial to the pubis and retracting the pectineus cranially. A second Hohmann retractor is placed caudal to the pubis, in the obturator foramen, and retracted caudally to provide adequate space for the osteotomy. Particular care should be taken when placing this caudal Hohmann retractor, as the obturator nerve and artery pass through the cranial border of the obturator foramen, along the caudal aspect of the isolated segment of pubic bone.
- The pubic osteotomy is performed using either an oscillating saw or Kerrison rongeurs. Some investigators recommend removing a segment of pubic bone, so that these areas of bone do not impinge during rotation of the acetabular segment. However, ostectomy is not necessary and rotation without impingement can be achieved with a single osteotomy.[33] The osteotomy should be performed immediately abaxial to the iliopubic eminence and immediately axial to the acetabulum (see **Fig. 6**). Osteotomies that are too far abaxial require cutting through substantially more bone, which is time consuming and unnecessary, and leaves the possibility of cutting into the acetabulum.[34] Conversely, osteotomies that are more axial can result in internal rotation of a substantial amount of pubis into the pelvic canal and risks impingement of intrapelvic structures, such as the urethra.[35,36] Whether an osteotomy or small ostectomy is performed, there is no

need to secure or reinforce the prepubic tendon. Subcutaneous tissues and skin are closed routinely.

Approach to the ilium

- A standard lateral approach to the ilium is performed with elevation of the deep and middle gluteal muscles from the ilium. Sharp transection of the middle gluteal from the cranial iliac spine is continued as far dorsally as necessary to allow adequate retraction of the middle gluteal dorsally and exposure to the dorsal ilial surface at the level of the planned osteotomy. Similarly, elevation of the iliacus muscle from the ventral aspect of the ilium can be performed to improve visualization of the ventral extent of the ilium. Such dissection often causes hemorrhage from severing a nutrient artery on the ventral aspect of the bone, which can be controlled with electrosurgery. Dissection and retraction on the medial aspect of the ilium is typically not necessary.
- The ilial osteotomy is usually performed immediately caudal to the junction with the sacrum, although it can be performed further caudal.[6] Great care should be taken to barely penetrate the transcortex to avoid damage to the obturator or sciatic nerves on the medial aspect of the ilium. The osteotomy should be oriented 10° to 30° from perpendicular to the long axis of the ilium, and closer to perpendicular to the long axis of the spine, in order to minimize any decrease in pelvic canal area while optimizing acetabular ventro-version (**Fig. 7**).[6,37,38] Bone-holding forceps are used to grasp and axially rotate the acetabular segment.
- The ilial bone plate that corresponds with the desired amount of rotation is selected and applied. The plate is typically secured to the caudal ilial segment first followed by attachment to the cranial segment. Adjunct implants, such as hemi-cerclage wire and/or ventral plate-screw constructs, may be applied (**Fig. 8**). If ischial hemi-cerclage wire was placed, it is now tightened.

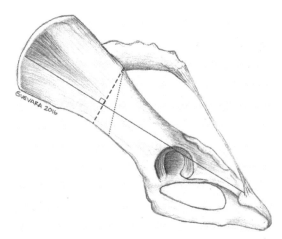

Fig. 7. Canine pelvis (lateral view) demonstrating different proposed osteotomies of the ilium. Previous iterations of the technique included performing the osteotomy perpendicular to the long axis of the pelvis (*dashed line*). More recent data suggests performing the osteotomy at an angle of 10° to 30° (usually 20°) to the long axis of the pelvis (*dotted line*).

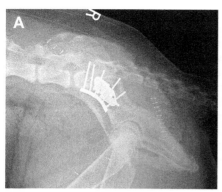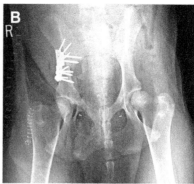

Fig. 8. (A) Lateral and (B) VD views, immediate postoperative unilateral DPO, of an 11-month-old castrated male Saint Bernard. A ventral bone plate was applied to mitigate the likelihood of implant failure in this giant breed. Healing was uncomplicated.

DEGREE OF ROTATION

The amount of acetabular ventro-version obtained at the time of surgery depends to a small degree on whether a TPO or DPO is performed but primarily on the implant used. Pelvic osteotomy implants are fabricated with a specific amount of rotation, typically 20°, 25°, 30°, and 40°.[38,39] Determining the amount of acetabular ventro-version that a surgeon should select is not entirely clear. Some investigators have suggested that the amount of rotation can be based on physical examination and should equal the AS plus 5° in order to prevent subluxation.[6] Similarly, intraoperative evaluation can be performed to determine whether Ortolani is resolved, and if not the degree of rotation can potentially be increased by substitution of a plate with a greater degree of inherent rotation. Although, achieving perfect screw hole alignment with the original screw holes following the increased rotation and replating may not be feasible.

Ex vivo studies have indicated that articular contact area progressively increases up to 30° of ventro-version but that contact area does not further increase with greater ventro-version.[40] Likewise, femoral head coverage increased significantly up to 20° of ventro-version but not more with additional ventro-version.[40] Those investigators suggested that increasing ventro-version beyond 20° did not seem to provide increasing benefit.[40] This work was corroborated by an in vivo study demonstrating that improvement in percent femoral head coverage and NA were the same for dogs treated with a 20° or 30° TPO.[41] Acetabular ventro-version beyond 30° may predispose to an increased potential for postoperative complications, such as reduced range of hip motion due to impingement of the dorsal acetabular rim on the femoral neck, medioventral subluxation of the femoral head, and narrowing of the pelvic canal.[40,41] In practice, variability in the amount of rotation used continues to depend on the individual surgeon and their chosen methodology for selecting the desired ventro-version.[32]

TRIPLE PELVIC OSTEOTOMY VERSUS DOUBLE PELVIC OSTEOTOMY

The TPO as described by Slocum and colleagues[5,14] is the best documented of the pelvic osteotomy techniques, and it is well established that the procedure effectively improves dorsal coverage of the femoral head and can provide good clinical results.[5,14,21] However, notable complication rates have also been reported with this procedure.[42–44] As a result, Haudiquet and Guillon[45] introduced the DPO, which is technically identical to the TPO as described by Slocum and colleagues[5,14] except that an ischial osteotomy is not performed. The ischial osteotomy is omitted because it is purported that retention of an intact ischium may provide a greater degree of immediate postoperative stability and, thus, improve comfort.[6] Likewise, it has been suggested that greater stability contributes to reduced implant loosening and fewer complications.[6] The rate of screw loosening in the one case series of dogs treated with DPO was substantially lower than that of earlier reports of TPO.[6,42–44] However, the decreased rate of screw loosening in the DPO case series may be attributable to advances in hardware and the use of locking plates. More recent reports on TPO using locking plates also detail a low rate of screw loosening.[32,34] Finally, an additional potential benefit of DPO is that pelvic canal width and geometry seem better maintained with DPO than with TPO, in which pelvic canal narrowing seems more common.[6,32,36] However, no direct comparisons of clinical application of TPO with DPO have been performed, so whether DPO truly provides greater immediate postoperative comfort, reduced implant loosening, and maintenance of pelvic width cannot be fully substantiated.

Although there may be benefits to leaving the ischium intact, there are also potential disadvantages of not performing an ischial osteotomy. Most notably, achieving acetabular ventro-version with DPO depends on plastic deformation including flattening of the pubic symphysis.[38] As a result, intraoperative rotation of the acetabular segment during DPO is subjectively more challenging than with TPO and particularly with bilateral procedures.[6] In addition, less acetabular ventro-version is achieved with DPO in comparison with TPO when the same preangled bone plate is used. An ex vivo study demonstrated that a 25° DPO results in a postoperative acetabular angle similar to that achieved with a 20° TPO.[38] Although achieving the desired amount of rotation during DPO presents additional difficulty, these challenges may be outweighed by potential benefits discussed earlier.

2.5 PELVIC OSTEOTOMY

The most recent variant in the current literature, the 2.5 PO, was described by Petazzoni and colleagues[39] in 2012. The investigators noted that TPO and DPO had similar clinical outcomes but that DPO was associated with a lower complication rate and better preserved pelvic geometry. During DPO, however, achieving ventro-version can be challenging and subjects the ischium to bending forces. Accordingly, postoperative ischial fracture has been reported and corresponds with subsequent narrowing of the pelvic canal.[6,39] In addition to standard pubic and ilial osteotomies, 2.5 PO uses an osteotomy of the dorsal cortex of the ischium in order to facilitate greater rotation of the acetabular segment. Use of an osteotomy on the dorsal cortex of the ischium may also minimize the tensile forces on the ischium and mitigate likelihood of ischial fracture.[39] However, it is feasible that the osteotomy may also weaken the bone and predispose to fracture. Subsequent fracture of the ischium that is not supported with hemicerclage wire could lead to pelvic canal narrowing. In addition, the procedure is comparatively complex and introduces additional technical challenges. No descriptions of clinical results using the 2.5 PO have been published.

IMPLANTS

Implants for pelvic osteotomy have evolved considerably since the procedure was first introduced. Early descriptions of implants range from a single cortical screw and hemicerclage wire to 4-hole, 3.5-mm dynamic compression (DCP) plate-screw constructs that were manually twisted and contoured intraoperatively.[5,46] The next generation of implants involved precontoured side-specific plates designed specifically for TPO.

More recent advances include similarly designed plates with angle-stable locking technology in an effort to improve implant stability and reduce screw loosening. Results from a cadaveric biomechanical evaluation demonstrated that significantly larger yield loads could be sustained when locking plate-screw constructs were used in conjunction with TPO.[47] Likewise, this study demonstrated that screw loosening was significantly reduced with the use of locking screws.[47] These ex vivo findings are supported by recent clinical case series demonstrating reduced rates of screw loosening in comparison with historical controls.[6,32,34] However, as a potential disadvantage, en bloc pullout of the screws from the caudal bone segment seems unique to the use of the locking plates and has been described in each of these case series as well.[6,32,34]

As an alternative method to decrease screw loosening, one prospective and one retrospective study provided data suggesting that maximal purchase into the sacrum of the most cranial screws would minimize loosening.[48,49] However, another report specified that screws placed into the sacrum were more likely to loosen.[50] Therefore, it is unclear whether placing screws in the sacrum is beneficial or detrimental. In addition, the risks of errantly violating the spinal canal should be considered, as does the need for obtaining sacral purchase if locking plates are used.[48] In the more recent clinical series that used locking plates, which had low rates of screw loosening, no sacral purchase was attempted.[6,32,34]

The adjunctive application of a ventrally applied bone plate is one more implant consideration. Application of such constructs has been shown to significantly increase construct stiffness and minimize screw loosening in a cadaveric study.[51] Further, application of a ventral plate reduced screw loosening in clinical patients.[52] As a result, application of a ventral plate is appealing and may be particularly beneficial in mature, active, or large- to giant-breed dogs in which the risk of implant loosening or failure is considered substantial. Although additional stability is provided, application of ventral plate-screw constructs can significantly increase the amount of surgical trauma via extension of the ilial approach, prolong anesthesia time, and increase costs. The use of ventral plates has also not been assessed in combination with the newer locking plates. Given the apparent decreased rates of screw loosening with newer locking plates, or DPO, the need for additional ventral fixation may be mitigated.

BILATERAL PROCEDURES

Hip dysplasia typically affects both coxofemoral joints, and many dogs affected by CHD may be candidates for bilateral treatment. Bilateral simultaneous procedures can be performed either with TPO or DPO (**Fig. 9**).[6,52] Benefits of this approach are that surgery is completed in a single anesthetic event, which is more efficient logistically and financially. In addition, simultaneous procedures mitigate the risk of progressive joint damage in an unoperated limb during the intervening period between staged procedures. However, bilateral simultaneous procedures have been associated with greater potential for complications, as higher rates of screw loosening with nonlocking constructs have been shown with bilateral rather than unilateral procedures.[52] If bilateral simultaneous procedures are to be performed, then one might consider the possible mechanical benefits of DPO (vs TPO), use of locking technology, and use of additional ventral plate fixation.

THE POSTOPERATIVE PERIOD
Postoperative Assessment and Patient Recovery

Radiographs should be taken immediately after surgery to evaluate technique and implant placement (see **Fig. 8**; **Fig. 10A**). Additionally, postoperative measurements

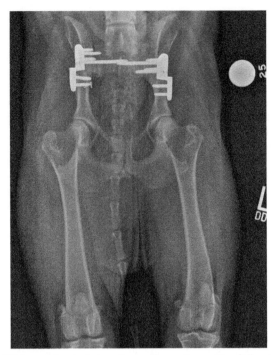

Fig. 9. Patient B: VD legs extended view, 3 months postoperative following bilateral simultaneous DPO. Note the improved femoral head coverage and maintenance of the pelvic geometry.

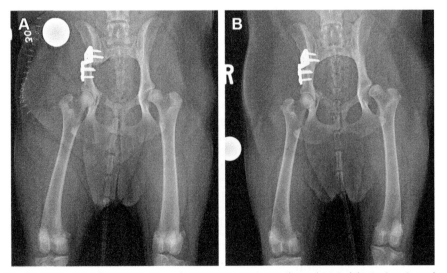

Fig. 10. Patient A: (*A*) VD view immediate postoperative unilateral DPO. (*B*) VD view 8 weeks postoperative showing complete osseous union; note progressive healing of the pubic osteotomy and progression of radiographic OA of the left coxofemoral joint with a circumferential head osteophyte.

for percent of femoral head coverage, Norberg angle, and pelvic width can be made for comparisons with preoperative status and to establish a baseline in comparison with subsequent radiographic examinations. The Ortolani test can be repeated immediately after surgery to confirm complete elimination or to subjectively assess the degree of improvement, with regard to angles of reduction and subluxation. Additional postoperative care is routine, the major components of which include provision of analgesia and activity modification until osseous union is obtained and documented radiographically (**Fig. 10**B). Physical rehabilitation may be beneficial, but evaluation of protocols specific to pelvic osteotomy have not been performed; readers are referred to references on canine physical rehabilitation.

OUTCOMES AND COMPLICATIONS OF PELVIC OSTEOTOMY

Current literature suggests that TPO and DPO procedures can improve function in young dogs with dysplastic hips. Both subjective and objective assessments suggest that dogs treated with TPO improve in their function.[33,53,54] Objective force plate data demonstrate a significant improvement in peak vertical force (PVF) in treated limbs[55] and acquisition of near-normal PVF values by 6 months following surgery.[54] However, despite improved function, the onset and/or progression of OA is not consistently prevented after TPO. Forty percent to 100% of dogs treated with TPO have documented radiographic progression of degenerative joint disease.[33,53,55] Further, postoperative complications have historically been prevalent. The most common include screw loosening and implant failure; however, reports of urethral impingement, over-rotation of the acetabular segment with femoral impingement and reduced abduction, pelvic canal narrowing, dysuria, and nerve damage have all been reported.[5,23,35,36,42–44,56] More recent reports seem to have fewer complications.[6,32,34] No recent comprehensive studies report on functional outcomes with objective kinetic data combined with data on complications, so it is challenging to succinctly summarize the effective outcomes and concurrent probability of complications with the advances in technique and implants over the last couple decades.

CURRENT CONTROVERSIES AND FUTURE CONSIDERATIONS FOR PELVIC OSTEOTOMY

Debate exists among surgeons as to whether pelvic osteotomies are successful, and there seems subjectively to be somewhat of a divide between surgeons who do pelvic osteotomies and those who do not believe in performing the procedure. The authors submit that whether the surgery is considered successful depends greatly on what the desired objectives of the procedure are and how one defines success. What data are available suggest that functional outcomes, whether assessed subjectively or objectively, are usually improved.[33,53–55] These data are limited in that the duration of follow-up is up to 2 years and extrapolation beyond that time is difficult. However, the evidence seems more convincing of clinical benefit rather than the contrary.

Although the data suggest pelvic osteotomy provides at least midterm functional benefit, the data also suggest that development or progression of OA is common.[33,53,55] Therefore, if the desired goals of the procedure are to prevent or mitigate progression of OA, it does not seem that pelvic osteotomies are widely successful. Arguments can be made against this statement, as previous studies have not always been highly selective and have either not included diagnostic arthroscopy to help exclude patients with preexisting cartilage pathology or have deliberately enrolled patients with evidence of substantial OA.[33,55] Accordingly, there are no studies that have reported on progression or onset of OA in a cohort of dogs that have all had diagnostic arthroscopy performed and in whom all dogs had either normal or minimal

(Outerbridge grade I) cartilage pathology. With that stated, the preponderance of studies show that a substantial portion of treated dogs show progression of OA as assessed radiographically.

In addition to considering the probability of success when determining whether to perform pelvic osteotomy, the financial costs and risk of complications must be weighed. Furthermore, the associated probability of success with other procedures, particularly nonsurgical management and salvage surgical procedures, including FHNE and THR, have to be considered. In this vein, a couple of different reasons may be suggested as to why many surgeons do not perform pelvic osteotomies. First, if the dog is sound, a surgeon may not believe in performing an invasive surgery with a risk of complications when a substantial proportion of such dogs may never demonstrate clinical signs of lameness or OA. This vantage point can be substantiated by the associated data correlating distraction indices and likelihood of lifetime OA development. Although dogs with moderate DIs often have a moderate likelihood of developing OA, they also have a moderate probability of not developing OA.[18,19] Second, if dogs are clinically dysfunctional, they often have at least some articular cartilage damage; the data support the conclusion that the OA will progress.[32,53,55] Accordingly, some surgeons would argue that if a pelvic osteotomy were performed in these dogs, there is a notable probability that OA will progress to the point that joint salvage surgery is ultimately needed, regardless of whether pelvic osteotomy is performed. In turn, some surgeons might conclude that one should wait and see whether such dogs become clinically affected enough to warrant joint salvage surgery and then perform either FHNE or THR at such time. There is sound logic to such reasoning.

Opposing vantage points held by surgeons in favor of performing pelvic osteotomies are numerous. As stated earlier, no studies have evaluated OA mitigation risk in dogs without notable preexisting cartilage pathology, and so the value of pelvic osteotomy in preventing OA progression in stringently selected patients without intra-articular pathology remains unclear. Second, some surgeons would argue that if a periarticular osteotomy improves function it is worth performing even if perfect stability and elimination of OA are not obtained.[6] There is a precedent for this logic, as tibial plateau leveling osteotomy does not consistently restore stifle stability or prevent progression of OA, yet evidence suggests it is clinically beneficial and is widely recommended for dogs with CCL rupture.[57–61] Third, as a general principle some surgeons would argue that a joint-preservation surgery, such as pelvic osteotomy, which preserves native cartilage and bone, is preferable to joint salvage surgeries that eliminate the native joint. Joint-salvage surgeries can be considered as last options for dogs with unrelenting pain and dysfunction and can be performed in animals that have already had pelvic osteotomy performed. Moreover, the cost, and possibly also the risk of complications, may be greater with THR than with pelvic osteotomy. Whether THR or pelvic osteotomies have a higher risk of complications depends on what studies are considered and are likely surgeon dependent.

There is logic to the different vantage points, and debate as to the value of pelvic osteotomies will likely continue into the foreseeable future. Additional data evaluating the benefit of such procedures could help with this decision-making process. Such study could take the form of a prospective randomized study comparing benefits in dogs managed conservatively and with pelvic osteotomy. Such study should include thorough staging of all dogs (or hips) including with physical examination, radiography, possibly CT, and arthroscopy and with stringent inclusion criteria. Dogs treated surgically and conservatively would need to be equivalent in these characteristics in order for comparisons to be robust. Outcomes would ideally include subjective assessments but also objective assessments, including kinetic force plate data, and would also be long-term with a follow-up of several years. Such study would represent a substantial investment of time and resources. Therefore, in the interim and for the foreseeable future, surgeons will have to make decisions on the value of pelvic osteotomy based on desired end goals of the procedure and the probability of success using those data that are currently available. The greatest degree of investment and improvement will likely continue to be in the realm of improvement in implants that potentially provide greater immediate stability and reduce complications associated with the procedure.

REFERENCES

1. Salter RB. Role of innominate osteotomy in the treatment of congenital dislocation and subluxation of the hip in the older child. J Bone Jt Surg Am Volume 1966; 48(7):1413–39.
2. Salter RB. The classic. Innominate osteotomy in the treatment of congenital dislocation and subluxation of the hip by Robert B. Salter, J. Bone Joint Surg. (Brit) 43B:3:518, 1961. Clin Orthop Relat Res 1978;(137):2–14.
3. Steel HH. Triple osteotomy of the innominate bone. J Bone Jt Surg Am Volume 1973;55(2):343–50.
4. Hohn RB, Janes JM. Pelvic osteotomy in the treatment of canine hip dysplasia. Clin Orthop Relat Res 1969;62:70–8.
5. Slocum B, Devine T. Pelvic osteotomy technique for axial rotation of the acetabular segment in dogs. J Am Anim Hosp Assoc 1986;22(3):331–8.
6. Vezzoni A, Boiocchi S, Vezzoni L, et al. Double pelvic osteotomy for the treatment of hip dysplasia in young dogs. Vet Comp Orthop Traumatol 2010;23(6):444–52.
7. Waxman AS, Robinson DA, Evans RB, et al. Relationship between objective and subjective assessment of limb function in normal dogs with an experimentally induced lameness. Vet Surg 2008;37(3):241–6.
8. Burton NJ, Owen MR, Colborne GR, et al. Can owners and clinicians assess outcome in dogs with fragmented medial coronoid process? Vet Comp Orthop Traumatol 2009;22(3):183–9.
9. Quinn MM, Keuler NS, Lu Y, et al. Evaluation of agreement between numerical rating scales, visual analogue scoring scales, and force plate gait analysis in dogs. Vet Surg 2007;36(4):360–7.
10. Lascelles BD, Roe SC, Smith E, et al. Evaluation of a pressure walkway system for measurement of vertical limb forces in clinically normal dogs. Am J Vet Res 2006; 67(2):277–82.
11. Light VA, Steiss JE, Montgomery RD, et al. Temporal-spatial gait analysis by use of a portable walkway system in healthy Labrador retrievers at a walk. Am J Vet Res 2010;71(9):997–1002.
12. Janssens LA, Beosier YM, Daems R. Triple pelvic osteotomy in dogs less than 12 kg in weight. Technical feasibility and short-term radiographic and clinical complications in fourteen hips. Vet Comp Orthop Traumatol 2010;23(6):453–8.
13. Chalman JA, Butler HC. Coxofemoral joint laxity and the Ortolani sign. J Am Anim Hosp Assoc 1985;21(5):671–6.
14. Slocum B, Slocum TD. Pelvic osteotomy for axial rotation of the acetabular segment in dogs with hip dysplasia. Vet Clin North America Small Anim Pract 1992;22(3):645–82.
15. Puerto DA, Smith GK, Gregor TP, et al. Relationships between results of the Ortolani method of hip joint palpation and distraction index, Norberg angle, and hip score in dogs. J Am Vet Med Assoc 1999;214(4):497–501.

16. Smith GK, Gregor TP, Rhodes WH, et al. Coxofemoral joint laxity from distraction radiography and its contemporaneous and prospective correlation with laxity, subjective score, and evidence of degenerative joint disease from conventional hip-extended radiography in dogs. Am J Vet Res 1993;54(7):1021–42.

17. Lust G, Williams AJ, Burton-Wurster N, et al. Joint laxity and its association with hip dysplasia in Labrador retrievers. Am J Vet Res 1993;54(12):1990–9.

18. Runge JJ, Kelly SP, Gregor TP, et al. Distraction index as a risk factor for osteoarthritis associated with hip dysplasia in four large dog breeds. J small Anim Pract 2010;51(5):264–9.

19. Smith GK, Mayhew PD, Kapatkin AS, et al. Evaluation of risk factors for degenerative joint disease associated with hip dysplasia in German shepherd dogs, golden retrievers, Labrador retrievers, and rottweilers. J Am Vet Med Assoc 2001;219(12):1719–24.

20. Trumpatori BJ, Mathews KG, Roe SR, et al. Radiographic anatomy of the canine coxofemoral joint using the dorsal acetabular rim (DAR) view. Vet Radiol Ultrasound 2003;44(5):526–32.

21. Slocum B, Devine TM. Dorsal acetabular rim radiographic view for evaluation of the canine hip. J Am Anim Hosp Assoc 1990;26(3):289–96.

22. Gold RM, Gregor TP, Huck JL, et al. Effects of osteoarthritis on radiographic measures of laxity and congruence in hip joints of Labrador retrievers. J Am Vet Med Assoc 2009;234(12):1549–54.

23. Tomlinson JL, Johnson JC. Quantification of measurement of femoral head coverage and Norberg angle within and among four breeds of dogs. Am J Vet Res 2000;61(12):1492–500.

24. Wang SI, Mathews KG, Robertson ID, et al. The effects of patient positioning and slice selection on canine acetabular angle assessment with computed tomography. Vet Radiol Ultrasound 2005;46(1):39–43.

25. Dueland RT, Adams WM, Patricelli AJ, et al. Canine hip dysplasia treated by juvenile pubic symphysiodesis. Part I: two year results of computed tomography and distraction index. Vet Comp Orthop Traumatol 2010;23(5):306–17.

26. Powers MY, Biery DN, Lawler DE, et al. Use of the caudolateral curvilinear osteophyte as an early marker for future development of osteoarthritis associated with hip dysplasia in dogs. J Am Vet Med Assoc 2004;225(2):233–7.

27. Szabo SD, Biery DN, Lawler DF, et al. Evaluation of a circumferential femoral head osteophyte as an early indicator of osteoarthritis characteristic of canine hip dysplasia in dogs. J Am Vet Med Assoc 2007;231(6):889–92.

28. Holsworth IG, Schulz KS, Kass PH, et al. Comparison of arthroscopic and radiographic abnormalities in the hip joints of juvenile dogs with hip dysplasia. J Am Vet Med Assoc 2005;227(7):1087–94.

29. Runge JJ, Biery DN, Lawler DF, et al. The effects of lifetime food restriction on the development of osteoarthritis in the canine shoulder. Vet Surg 2008;37(1):102–7.

30. Fortrie RR, Verhoeven G, Broeckx B, et al. Intra- and interobserver agreement on radiographic phenotype in the diagnosis of canine hip dysplasia. Vet Surg 2015; 44(4):467–73.

31. Lopez MJ, Lewis BP, Swaab ME, et al. Relationships among measurements obtained by use of computed tomography and radiography and scores of cartilage microdamage in hip joints with moderate to severe joint laxity of adult dogs. Am J Vet Res 2008;69(3):362–70.

32. Rose SA, Bruecker KA, Petersen SW, et al. Use of locking plate and screws for triple pelvic osteotomy. Vet Surg 2012;41(1):114–20.

33. Manley PA, Adams WM, Danielson KC, et al. Long-term outcome of juvenile pubic symphysiodesis and triple pelvic osteotomy in dogs with hip dysplasia. J Am Vet Med Assoc 2007;230(2):206–10.

34. Rose SA, Peck JN, Tano CA, et al. Effect of a locking triple pelvic osteotomy plate on screw loosening in 26 dogs. Vet Surg 2012;41(1):156–62.

35. Dudley RM, Wilkens BE. Urethral obstruction as a complication of staged bilateral triple pelvic osteotomy. J Am Anim Hosp Assoc 2004;40(2):162–4.

36. Papadopoulos G, Tommasini Degna M. Two cases of dysuria as a complication of single-session bilateral triple pelvic osteotomy. J small Anim Pract 2006;47(12): 741–3.

37. Graehler RA, Weigel JP, Pardo AD. The effects of plate type, angle of iliac osteotomy, and degree of axial rotation on the structural anatomy of the pelvis. Vet Surg 1994;23(1):13–20.

38. Punke JP, Fox DB, Tomlinson JL, et al. Acetabular ventroversion with double pelvic osteotomy versus triple pelvic osteotomy: a cadaveric study in dogs. Vet Surg 2011;40(5):555–62.

39. Petazzoni M, Tamburro R, Nicetto T, et al. Evaluation of the dorsal acetabular coverage obtained by a modified triple pelvic osteotomy (2.5 pelvic osteotomy): an ex vivo study on a cadaveric canine codel. Vet Comp Orthop Traumatol 2012; 25(5):385–9.

40. Dejardin LM, Perry RL, Arnoczky SP. The effect of triple pelvic osteotomy on the articular contact area of the hip joint in dysplastic dogs: an in vitro experimental study. Vet Surg 1998;27(3):194–202.

41. Tomlinson JL, Cook JL. Effects of degree of acetabular rotation after triple pelvic osteotomy on the position of the femoral head in relationship to the acetabulum. Vet Surg 2002;31(4):398–403.

42. Remedios AM, Fries CL. Implant complications in 20 triple pelvic osteotomies. Vet Comp Orthop Traumatol 1993;6(4):202–7.

43. Hosgood G, Lewis DD. Retrospective evaluation of fixation complications of 49 pelvic osteotomies in 36 dogs. J Small Anim Pract 1993;34(3):123–30.

44. Koch DA, Hazewinkel HA, Nap RC, et al. Radiographic evaluation and comparison of plate fixation after triple pelvic osteotomy in 32 dogs with hip dysplasia. Vet Comp Orthop Traumatol 1993;6(1):9–15.

45. Haudiquet P, Guillon JF. Radiographic evaluation of double pelvic osteotomy versus triple pelvic osteotomy in the dog: an in vitro experimental study. In: Vezzoni A, Innes J, Lepage O, editors. 14th ESVOT Congress Proceedings, Munich, Germany, 10-14 September 2008. The cutting edge in veterinary orthopaedics CE. Cremona (Italy): European Society of Veterinary Orthopaedics and Traumatology; 2008. p. 85–6.

46. Schrader SC. Triple osteotomy of the pelvis as a treatment for canine hip dysplasia. J Am Vet Med Assoc 1981;178(1):39–44.

47. Case JB, Dean C, Wilson DM, et al. Comparison of the mechanical behaviors of locked and nonlocked plate/screw fixation applied to experimentally induced rotational osteotomies in canine ilia. Vet Surg 2012;41(1):103–13.

48. Whelan MF, McCarthy RJ, Boudrieau RJ, et al. Increased sacral screw purchase minimizes screw loosening in canine triple pelvic osteotomy. Vet Surg 2004;33(6): 609–14.

49. Simmons S, Johnson AL, Schaeffer DJ. Risk factors for screw migration after triple pelvic osteotomy. J Am Anim Hosp Assoc 2001;37(3):269–73.

50. Doornink MT, Nieves MA, Evans R. Evaluation of ilial screw loosening after triple pelvic osteotomy in dogs: 227 cases (1991-1999). J Am Vet Med Assoc 2006; 229(4):535–41.

51. Fitch RB, Hosgood G, Staatz A. Biomechanical evaluation of triple pelvic osteotomy with and without additional ventral plate stabilization. Vet Comp Orthop Traumatol 2002;15(3):145–9.

52. Fitch RB, Kerwin S, Hosgood G, et al. Radiographic evaluation and comparison of triple pelvic osteotomy with and without additional ventral plate stabilization in forty dogs - Part 1. Vet Comp Orthop Traumatol 2002;15(3):164–71.

53. Rasmussen LM, Kramek BA, Lipowitz AJ. Preoperative variables affecting long-term outcome of triple pelvic osteotomy for treatment of naturally developing hip dysplasia in dogs. J Am Vet Med Assoc 1998;213(1):80–5.

54. McLaughlin RM Jr, Miller CW, Taves CL, et al. Force plate analysis of triple pelvic osteotomy for the treatment of canine hip dysplasia. Vet Surg 1991;20(5):291–7.

55. Johnson AL, Smith CW, Pijanowski GJ, et al. Triple pelvic osteotomy: effect on limb function and progression of degenerative joint disease. J Am Anim Hosp Assoc 1998;34(3):260–4.

56. Tong K, Hayashi K. Obturator nerve impingement as a severe late complication of bilateral triple pelvic osteotomy. Vet Comp Orthop Traumatol 2012;25(1):67–70.

57. Duerr FM, Martin KW, Rishniw M, et al. Treatment of canine cranial cruciate ligament disease. A survey of ACVS Diplomates and primary care veterinarians. Vet Comp Orthop Traumatol 2014;27(6):478–83.

58. Kim SE, Lewis DD, Pozzi A. Effect of tibial plateau leveling osteotomy on femorotibial subluxation: in vivo analysis during standing. Vet Surg 2012;41(4):465–70.

59. Johnson K, Lanz O, Elder S, et al. The effect of stifle angle on cranial tibial translation following tibial plateau leveling osteotomy: an in vitro experimental analysis. Can Vet J 2011;52(9):961–6.

60. Au KK, Gordon-Evans WJ, Dunning D, et al. Comparison of short- and long-term function and radiographic osteoarthrosis in dogs after postoperative physical rehabilitation and tibial plateau leveling osteotomy or lateral fabellar suture stabilization. Vet Surg 2010;39(2):173–80.

61. Wucherer KL, Conzemius MG, Evans R, et al. Short-term and long-term outcomes for overweight dogs with cranial cruciate ligament rupture treated surgically or nonsurgically. J Am Vet Med Assoc 2013;242(10):1364–72.

Femoral Head and Neck Excision

Tisha A.M. Harper, DVM, MS, CCRP

KEYWORDS

- Femoral head and neck excision • Femoral head and neck ostectomy
- Femoral head ostectomy • Excision arthroplasty • FHO

KEY POINTS

- Femoral head and neck excision should be used judiciously and should not be used in dysplastic patients without clinical signs.
- Femoral head and neck excision should only be used as a salvage procedure after all other therapies have failed and should not be overused in patients if the coxofemoral joint can be restored.
- Caution should be used when considering femoral head and neck excision in immature patients with hip dysplasia because improvement in hind limb function may occur as the patient matures.
- The patient should be thoroughly evaluated for concurrent orthopedic or neurologic conditions before performing a femoral head and neck excision.
- Complete removal of the femoral head and neck and aggressive postoperative physical therapy are necessary to maximize function postoperatively.

INTRODUCTION

Hip dysplasia is a common orthopedic disease seen in large and giant breeds of dogs.[1–5] It has also been described in cats.[6,7] In dogs, the disease is characterized by laxity of the soft tissues of the hip, resulting in instability and eventually abnormal growth and development of the coxofemoral joint.[2,3,8] Malformation of the femoral head and acetabulum leads to the development of osteoarthritis and pain in the coxofemoral joint.[2,8] In immature patients, the pain associated with hip dysplasia is primarily due to the continuous luxation or subluxation of the femoral head.[2,9] Lateral displacement of the femoral head results in an increase in the joint reaction force and also concentrates this force over a smaller area, directing the contact between the femoral head and acetabulum between 10 o'clock and 2 o'clock.[2,3,8] This causes stress and overloading of the dorsal acetabular rim, leading to the development of

Disclosure Statement: The author has nothing to disclose.
Department of Veterinary Clinical Medicine, University of Illinois College of Veterinary Medicine, 1008 West Hazelwood Drive, Urbana, IL 61802, USA
E-mail address: taharper@illinois.edu

Vet Clin Small Anim 47 (2017) 885–897
http://dx.doi.org/10.1016/j.cvsm.2017.03.002
vetsmall.theclinics.com

microfractures in the developing trabecular cancellous bone of the acetabulum.[3,8,9] Loss of congruity between the articular surfaces of the femoral head and acetabulum also occurs secondary to the laxity in the periarticular soft tissues.[3,8] The constant displacement of the femoral head can also cause stretching of the fibrous joint capsule, as well as tension and tearing of the sensory nerves of the fibrous periosteum. Disruption of Sharpey's fibers and stimulation of the periosteum can lead to pain and osteophyte formation on the acetabulum and femoral neck.[3,8,10,11] In immature patients, the pain due to extreme joint laxity is manifested as exercise intolerance or reduced exercise tolerance, bunny hopping, difficulty rising after rest, and intermittent or continuous lameness.[1,2,8,9] In older patients, pain and dysfunction are secondary to the development of osteoarthritis, which is manifested as atrophy of the hind limb musculature, difficulty rising, stiffness in the pelvic limbs, and reluctance to walk, run, or jump.[2,9,11] Cats seem to tolerate laxity in the hips better than dogs and subluxation does not seem to be a primary component of the disease process.[6] Osteoarthritis is also seen at comparatively higher distraction index values.[6]

Femoral head and neck excision (FHNE) is a common surgical procedure performed on the coxofemoral joint.[12] It was originally described and used to treat septic arthritis of the hip in human patients and was then adapted and adopted by veterinary surgeons.[13] The aim of this procedure is to limit bony contact between the femoral head and acetabulum and allow formation of a false joint (pseudoarthrosis) made up of dense fibrous tissue.[9,12,14] Remodeling of the acetabulum and proximal femur may continue for years following surgery.[15] FHNE is commonly performed to relieve pain secondary to degenerative joint disease, thus improving comfort and function.[4,12,16] The pain is relieved by elimination of bony contact between the femur and pelvis.[8] FHNE is considered a salvage procedure.[12] The goal is to improve the patient's quality of life by allowing pain-free movement during moderate activity.

INDICATIONS

Treatment of hip dysplasia can either be directed at providing pain relief or preventing or lessening the amount of future osteoarthritis.[1,8,9,17] FHNE can address both goals. It can provide immediate pain relief in patients with debilitating coxofemoral osteoarthritis that is unresponsive to nonsurgical methods. Also, if the integrity of the hip has been compromised; for example, highly comminuted acetabular fracture, and primary repair is not feasible, FHNE will prevent the development of osteoarthritis in the future as there is no longer an intact diarthroidal joint.[8] Factors that must be considered before deciding whether or not to perform FHNE include

- Age of the patient
- Severity of clinical signs
- Physical examination and radiographic findings
- Presence of other orthopedic diseases
- Breed and temperament
- Expected patient performance
- Financial constraints of the client
- Skill of the surgeon
- Internal fixation devices available.

Management of hip dysplasia should be based on individual needs of the patient. There are other surgical procedures that will result in more predictable outcomes; for example, pelvic osteotomies in immature patients or total hip replacement in mature patients. However, if other surgical procedures are precluded by financial constraints, other comorbidities, size, age, or excessive laxity, FHNE may be considered. FHNE should not be done without informed consent of the client.

Specific indications for FHNE[17–19] include

- Chronic or recurrent coxofemoral luxation
- Severe coxofemoral osteoarthritis
- Comminuted or complicated femoral head, neck, or acetabular fractures
- Avascular necrosis of the femoral head
- Failed total hip replacement.

There are no specific weight guidelines for FHNE. The procedure can be performed in small animal patients of any size.[7,20] Generally, smaller patients tend to have better results than larger patients.[12,18,20–22] FHNE is often chosen by pet owners because of financial constraints and the potential for severe complications associated with total hip replacement. In the past, FHNE was also used in patients with pathologic conditions of the coxofemoral joint but were too small for total hip replacement. With the advent of smaller prosthetic hip implants, this is less of a concern, though micro and nano hip replacements are not as widely available as total hip replacements for larger patients.[23–26] Many immature patients with clinical signs of hip dysplasia will improve with maturity; therefore, careful case selection is important.[1] In immature patients with mild disease, pet owners should be encouraged to follow prescribed conservative management strategies.[9] It is not uncommon to have dogs with hip dysplasia that have clinically been doing well, present with sudden or progressive hind limb lameness. Many of these pets have other orthopedic or neurologic problems; for example, cranial cruciate ligament rupture or lumbosacral disease.[16] Therefore, before surgery, thorough orthopedic and neurologic examinations should be performed to determine if the discomfort or lameness is truly attributable to hip dysplasia.

TECHNIQUE AND PROCEDURE
Preparation and Patient Positioning

The patient is placed in lateral recumbency with the affected limb uppermost. The hair should be clipped from dorsal midline to just distal to the stifle or the clip can be extended to the hock. A hanging limb technique is used for limb preparation.[27] Draping should be performed to allow manipulation of the limb during surgery.

Approach

Anatomy of the bones and soft tissue of the hip should be reviewed before surgery.[28] Access to the coxofemoral joint to perform FHNE can be gained by using either a craniolateral approach or a ventral approach.[27] Exposure of the joint is much more limited using the ventral approach.[27] The approach to the craniodorsal aspect of the hip using a craniolateral incision is more common and has been well described in the dog and cat.[11,27] Once the joint capsule has been incised and the femoral head is visible, the following steps should be performed to complete FHNE.

Technique and Procedure

- The hip must be luxated to facilitate FHNE. In pets with severe chronic osteoarthritis, the ligament of the head of the femur is often torn or worn away and is not present at the time of surgery; therefore, the hip is readily luxated.[4] If the ligament of the head of the femur is intact, it must be transected. This can be done by using a femoral ligament cutter (Hatt Spoon) or curved Mayo scissors placed into the joint. Subluxation of the femoral head facilitates placement of these instruments into the joint. This can be achieved by placing bone-holding forceps on the greater trochanter and applying lateral and distal traction of the proximal femur.

- Exposure of the cranial surface of the proximal femur is necessary to perform the ostectomy (**Fig. 1**). The limb is therefore externally rotated 90° so that the cranial surface of the femur is parallel to the operating table and the patella is pointing toward the ceiling. Hohmann retractors placed intracapsularly, ventral and caudal to the femoral neck provide leverage, aid in exposure, help to protect the soft tissues, and help to stabilize the femoral head and neck. The caudal retractor is typically placed in the trochanteric fossa between the deep gluteal muscle and the bone.

- The line of transection should be identified at the junction of the femoral neck and the femoral metaphysis and should be performed using an osteotome or an oscillating saw. The cut should begin just medial to the greater trochanter proximally; that is, at the most lateral extent of the trochanteric fossa and directed caudally and medially to end just proximal to or bisecting the lesser trochanter distally.[12] Once the osteotome or saw is placed on the ostectomy line, the handle of the saw or osteotome should be directed toward the animal's trunk; that is, parallel to the sagittal plane of the thigh.[8] This will avoid leaving a shelf of bone on the caudal femoral neck that could potentially rub on the acetabular rim, preventing the formation of fibrous tissue between the bones (pseudoarthrosis).[8] When performing the ostectomy, care should be taken to prevent excessive damage to perifemoral soft tissues, particularly along the caudal aspect of the femur in the region of the sciatic nerve.

- Once the ostectomy is complete, bone-holding forceps can be used to grasp the femoral head and remaining soft tissue attachments; for example, the joint capsule should be incised to allow complete removal of the femoral head and neck.

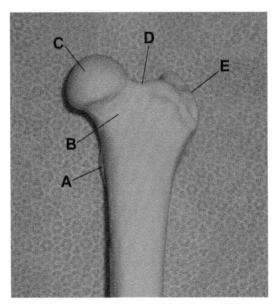

Fig. 1. Important landmarks to note on the cranial surface of the proximal femur before resection of the femoral head and neck: (A) lesser trochanter, (B) femoral neck, (C) femoral head, (D) trochanteric fossa, (E) greater trochanter.

- The cut surface of the femoral metaphysis is then palpated for any irregularities. The most common finding is a shelf of femoral neck left on the caudal surface of the femur due to the osteotome or saw being placed perpendicular to the surgery table. The limb should also be moved proximally and distally to feel for any crepitus. Remove any rough edges with a rongeur or a bone rasp. This is facilitated by further external rotation of the limb to expose the caudal femoral cut surface. Excessive osteophyte formation on the dorsal acetabular rim should also be debrided.[8]

Suture the joint capsule over the acetabulum, if possible, using simple interrupted or mattress sutures, using absorbable suture material. The surgical site is then closed using standard methods.[27] Postoperative radiographs should be taken following surgery to determine if sufficient femoral neck has been removed and that no fractures of the greater trochanter or femur are observed.[4,16]

In the author's experience, the following tips are helpful to ensure a successful procedure:

- Ensure that the ligament of the femoral head is completely transected. Often it is only partially transected and complete luxation of the femoral head is not achieved. This makes appropriate positioning of the femur for the ostectomy difficult.
- If FHNE is performed for traumatic coxofemoral luxation in a normal hip, attempt to reduce the hip before making the surgical approach. This helps to maintain normal anatomy during dissection.
- Ensure a 90° angle of rotation of the limb so that it is perpendicular to its original axis; that is, the patella is pointing to the ceiling. If the limb is not appropriately positioned and allowed to rotate internally, there will be inadequate bone removal at the caudal aspect of the femoral neck. An assistant should maintain the correct position of the limb.
- Do not be afraid to reflect the vastus lateralis distally off the femoral neck to allow appropriate exposure of the femoral neck.
- In older patients with moderate to severe osteoarthritis, there may be significant osteophyte production and remodeling of the femoral neck, making identification of the trochanteric fossa and the delineation between the greater trochanter and the femoral head and neck difficult. This can either lead to inadvertent transection of the greater trochanter or incomplete removal of the femoral neck. Use of a rongeur to remove osteophytes present in the trochanteric fossa will help to better define the femoral neck (**Figs. 2–4**).
- An oscillating saw is preferred over an osteotome because it provides the smoothest and most accurate cut[12,17] (**Fig. 5**). An osteotome should probably be avoided in pets with chronic disuse atrophy of the limb because the bone is often osteopenic and can shatter easily, potentially leading to fracture of the greater trochanter or femoral shaft.
- Always over-rotate the limb externally after the ostectomy to inspect the cut surface of the bone. Ensure that it is smooth. A bone rasp or rongeur can be used to smooth the ostectomy site.
- Consider removal of the dorsal acetabular rim, particularly in dogs with chronic hip dysplasia in which there may be significant osteophyte formation along the dorsal acetabular rim.

FHNE can be performed bilaterally, separated by an interval of 8 to 10 weeks.[8] It can also be done simultaneously during a single anesthetic episode for the treatment of

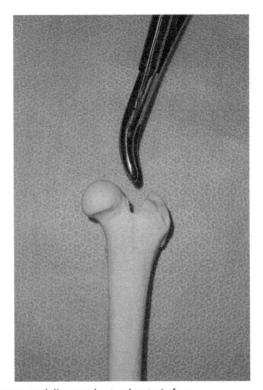

Fig. 2. Use of rongeurs to delineate the trochanteric fossa.

severe bilateral hip dysplasia.[4] In a study evaluating the clinical outcome in 15 dogs, ranging in weight from 19 to 30.9 kg, undergoing bilateral FHNE to treat severe bilateral hip dysplasia, 4 were walking without assistance on the second postoperative day and all dogs were walking within 4 days. Owners graded the results of surgery as good to excellent, and stronger jumping, better use of stairs, and greater exercise tolerance over time were noted.[4] Presumably these dogs were so severely affected by their

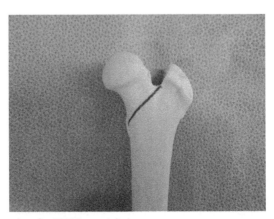

Fig. 3. Line of resection for FHNE, cranial view.

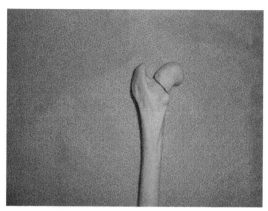

Fig. 4. Line of resection for FHNE, caudal view.

disease that their quality of life was significantly improved with bilateral surgery. Possible advantages of simultaneous bilateral FHNE include shorter overall recovery time, decreased number of anesthetic episodes, more cost-effective for the owner, and symmetry in the recovering limbs.[4]

COMPLICATIONS AND MANAGEMENT

General complications associated with surgery may be seen; that is, anesthetic and surgical site infection. Complications specific to FHNE surgery include

- Shortening of the limb, which may be secondary to tilting of the pelvis and stifle flexion[7,18,29]
- Damage to or entrapment of the sciatic nerve[30]
- Patellar luxation[18,19]
- Muscle atrophy[4,7,29]
- Decreased range of motion of the hip, particularly on extension[7,18]
- Continued pain, lameness, and reduced exercise tolerance.[7,18,20]

POSTOPERATIVE CARE

Contrary to postoperative care for many orthopedic procedures, restricted activity and strict cage rest following FHNE surgery are contraindicated. These patients must be encouraged to use the limb as early and as frequently after surgery as possible, otherwise the fibrous tissue that forms during the postoperative period will be restrictive and severely limit range of motion of the coxofemoral joint. Physical therapy is therefore critical to maximize function in the postoperative period. Passive range of motion exercises and walking should begin immediately postoperatively, moving on to further active exercises within 2 to 3 weeks. **Table 1** outlines a general rehabilitation program that can be used following FHNE. However, protocols that are patient-specific are preferred, particularly in patients with other orthopedic disease or comorbidities. Appropriate, often multimodal, analgesia in the postoperative period is critical to ensure patient comfort and to facilitate physical therapy.

Note: If FHNE is to be performed as an elective procedure; that is, for most hip dysplasia patients, the author encourages pet owners to do physical therapy before surgery, particularly in patients with significant muscle atrophy. These patients often

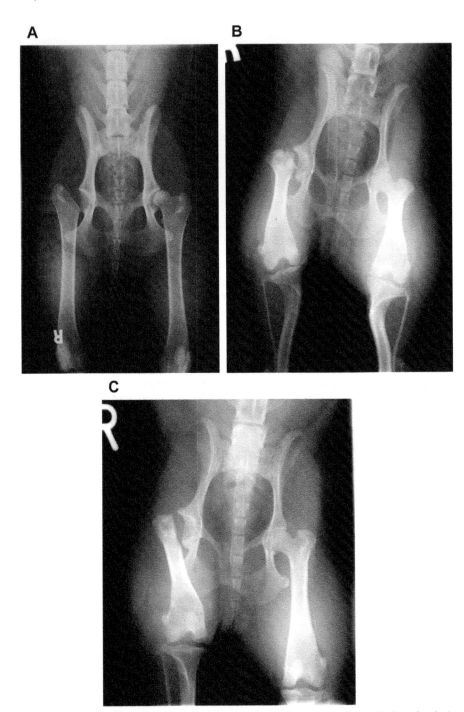

Fig. 5. Ventrodorsal radiographs following FHNE. (*A*) In a young dog with hip dysplasia, note complete removal of the femoral head and neck. The lesser trochanter was preserved. The resection was performed using an oscillating saw. (*B*) Incomplete removal of the femoral neck in a dog with avascular necrosis of the femoral head. (*C*) Revision of FHNE of dog in (*B*).

Table 1
Physical rehabilitation following femoral head and neck ostectomy

All Treatments q12h	Day 1 to Day 14	Day 15 to Day 24	Day 25 Until Healed	Healed to Return to Function
Heat Therapy	—	10 min	10 min	—
Massage	5 min	5 min	5 min	—
Passive range of motion (repetitions)	15[a]	15[a]	15[a]	15[a]
Electrical stimulation[b]	10 min	10 min	10 min	10 min
Therapeutic exercise: total time	15 min	25 min	30 min	25–45 min
Walk or land treadmill	5 min	10 min	10 min	>10 min
Balancing	+	+	+	+
Obstacles	+	+	+	+
Weaving	+	+	+	+
Circles	—	+	+	+
Hills	—	+	+	+
Stairs	—	—	+	+
Jog or run	—	—	+	+
Underwater treadmill	10 min	5 min	20 min	>25 min
Swimming	5 min	—	15 min	20 min
Cryotherapy	15 min	15 min	15 min	PRN

+, perform modality; PRN, as needed.
[a] Perform passive range of motion to all joints of the affected limb.
[b] Electrical stimulation to be performed on the semimembranosus or semitendinosus muscle groups in patients with muscle atrophy.
From Fossum TW. Diseases of the joints. Small animal surgery. Chapter 34. 4th edition. St Louis (MO): Elsevier Mosby; 2012; with permission.

do better after surgery if muscle mass and tone are improved before the procedure. This is based on the premise that the pain can be well controlled with analgesics to facilitate physical therapy.

OUTCOMES

Criteria that have been used to assess functional outcome following FHNE include range of motion; degree and direction of displacement of the femur, stifle, and hock angles; muscle mass; kinetic and kinematic analyses; radiographic findings; and goniometric measurements.[29,31] Many studies cite better postoperative results in dogs weighing less than 18 to 20 kg.[7,20,21] It is thought that dogs weighing greater than 20 kg have poorer results following FHNE because their heavier mass tends to increase bony contact between the cut surface of the femoral metaphysis and the acetabular rim and pelvis.[21] However, any pet with debilitating osteoarthritis in the coxofemoral joint undergoing a correctly performed FHNE can be expected to have improved limb function and quality of life following surgery compared with not performing surgery.[9,18,19] Other factors that can influence postoperative outcome include age, temperament, activity, surgical technique, postoperative physical therapy, and the severity of muscle atrophy at the time of surgery.[5,7,12,17,32,33] The biomechanics of the hind limb change following FHNE because the femoral head no longer articulates with the acetabulum and a fibrous false joint is present. This results in a change in gait due to limb-shortening, dorsal displacement of the femur, muscle atrophy, and decreased stifle and hock angles, as well as restricted extension of the hip.[7,17,18] Return to maximal function following FHNE can take as long as 6 months[5] and depends on the chronicity of disease before surgery. Patients with chronic disease seem to return to function more slowly than those with acute lameness; for example, patients with femoral neck fracture that already have good muscle mass.[9,20,34] Aggressive pain management and aggressive physical therapy are therefore critical in the early postoperative period to allow early use of the limb.[5] Long-term problems that can be seen include persistent lameness, discomfort after excessive exercise, stiffness in cold weather, difficulty jumping and climbing stairs, and muscle atrophy.[5,15,18,32,33,35] Although most information in the literature is focused on the outcome of FHNE in dogs, cats have been reported to have good-to-excellent medium-term to long-term functional outcome after adequately performed FHNE.[7,19,36] Generally, outcomes are difficult to compare between studies due to several confounding factors, including owner evaluation of outcome, lack of objective measures, use of normal dogs, variations in surgical technique, differences in follow-up times, differences in postoperative physical therapy, and lack of postoperative radiographs in some cases.

CURRENT CONTROVERSIES AND FUTURE CONSIDERATIONS

Bone-on-bone contact between the femur and acetabulum or pelvis is one of the factors thought to play an important role in outcome following FHNE. The bone-on-bone contact is thought to be a significant cause of pain, discomfort, and an unwillingness to use the operated limb, particularly during the early postoperative period,[7,18] especially in large and giant breeds of dogs.[12,21,22] This fueled many studies looking at techniques for interposition of soft tissue between the cut surface of the femur and the acetabulum to decrease bony contact.[14,19,21,22,37–39] The most commonly used tissues are the joint capsule, deep gluteal muscle flap, and either full or partial-thickness biceps femoris muscle sling.[7,14,21,22,37] The partial thickness biceps sling has been shown to provide more coverage of the femoral ostectomy site compared with the gluteal muscle flap.[37] Although the biceps femoris muscle sling has been shown in some studies to result in pain-free ambulation in larger dogs compared with those with excision arthroplasty of the femoral head and neck alone,[21,40] other studies showed no difference in outcome regardless of technique used to achieve FHNE.[29,33,38,39] Interpretation of the results of some of these studies is difficult because some procedures were performed on normal dogs.[14,29,37] Also, the significance of bone-on-bone contact on long-term function is uncertain.[5] The use of muscle slings or flaps seems to have fallen out of favor and their routine use is no longer recommended.[17] Their use can be considered in patients with severe muscle atrophy and in revision surgeries.[17]

FHNE was, in the past, considered a nonreversible procedure. Revisions following failed FHNE with total hip replacement have now been reported in both dogs and cats.[30,41] Although the choice of FHNE versus total hip replacement is often made based on financial considerations and the potential associated complications, revision may be a viable alternative in select cases.[30,41]

There are few objective studies looking at the effect of removal of the lesser trochanter. In 2 long-term studies, removal of the lesser trochanter did not seem to have an effect on outcome following FHNE.[7,20] However, maintaining the entire lesser trochanter or a portion of it was shown to result in significantly higher vertical impulses at a walk and peak vertical force at a trot.[34] Muscle attachments at the lesser trochanter are likely important for postoperative limb mobility and stability and it is the author's preference to maintain the lesser trochanter or at least a portion of it during FHNE.

SUMMARY

FHNE is a simple, relatively inexpensive, surgical procedure that can be used to alleviate pain in the coxofemoral joint. Proper surgical technique, appropriate postoperative analgesia, and aggressive postoperative physical therapy are necessary to maximize function in the limb. The procedure should be reserved for patients with debilitating osteoarthritis of the coxofemoral joint that is unresponsive to nonsurgical management and for which other surgical therapies are not options. FHNE may also be used in patients with acute injuries to the coxofemoral joint in which the integrity of the joint cannot be restored. Significant functional changes will occur in the hind limb following FHNE surgery.

REFERENCES

1. Barr ARS, Denny HR, Gibbs C. Clinical hip dysplasia in growing dogs: the long-term results of conservative management. J Small Anim Pract 1987;28:243–52.
2. Smith GK, Karbe GT, Agnello KA, et al. Pathogenesis, diagnosis, and control of canine hip dysplasia. In: Tobias KM, Johnston SA, editors. Veterinary surgery small animal. St Louis (MO): Elsevier Saunders; 2012. p. 824–48.
3. Riser WH. The dysplastic hip joint: its radiographic and histologic development. J Am Vet Radiol Soc 1973;14:35–50.
4. Rawson EA, Aronsohn MG, Burk RL. Simultaneous bilateral femoral head and neck ostectomy for the treatment of canine hip dysplasia. J Am Anim Hosp Assoc 2005;41(3):166–70.
5. Plante J, Dupuis J, Beauregard G, et al. Long-term results of conservative treatment, excision arthroplasty and triple pelvic osteotomy for the treatment of hip dysplasia in the immature dog: Part 1 Radiographic and physical results. Vet Comp Orthop Traumatol 1997;10:101–10.
6. Perry K. Feline hip dysplasia: A challenge to recognise and treat. J Feline Med Surg 2016;18(3):203–18.
7. Off W, Matis U. Excision arthroplasty of the hip joint in dogs and cats. Clinical, radiographic, and gait analysis findings from the Department of Surgery, Veterinary Faculty of the Ludwig-Maximilians-University of Munich, Germany. Vet Comp Orthop Traumatol 2010;23(5):297–305.
8. Piermattei DL, Flo GL, DeCamp CE. The hip joint. Handbook of small animal orthopedics and fracture repair. 4th edition. St Louis (MO): Saunders Elsevier; 2006. p. 475–511.
9. Fossum TW. Diseases of the joints. Small animal surgery. 4th edition. St Louis (MO): Elsevier Mosby; 2012. p. 1305–16.
10. Krotscheck U, Tohundter T. Pathogenesis of hip dysplasia. In: Bojrab MJ, Monnet E, editors. Mechanisms of disease in small animal surgery. 3rd edition. Jackson (WY): Teton New Media; 2012. p. 636–45.
11. Schulz KS, Dejardin LM. Surgical treatment of canine hip dysplasia. In: Slatter D, editor. Textbook of small animal surgery. 3rd edition. Philadelphia: W B Saunders; 2002. p. 2029–59.
12. Prostredny JM. Excision arthroplasty of the femoral head and neck. In: Bojrab MJ, editor. Current techniques in small animal surgery. 5th edition. Jackson (WY): Teton New Media; 2014. p. 1048–52.
13. Girdlestone GR. Acute pyogenic arthritis of the hip. Lancet 1943;241(6):419–21.

14. Lewis DD, Bellah JR, McGavin MD, et al. Postoperative examination of the biceps femoris muscle sling used in excision of the femoral head and neck in dogs. Vet Surg 1988;17(5):269–77.
15. Duff R, Campbell JR. Radiographic appearance and clinical progress after excision arthroplasty of the canine hip. J Small Anim Pract 1978;19(8):439–49.
16. Lippincott CL. Femoral head and neck excision in the management of canine hip dysplasia. Vet Clin North Am Small Anim Pract 1992;22(3):721–37.
17. Roush JK. Surgical therapy of canine hip dysplasia. In: Tobias KM, Johnston SA, editors. Veterinary surgery small animal. St Louis (MO): Elsevier Saunders; 2012. p. 849–64.
18. Duff R, Campbell JR. Long term results of excision arthroplasty of the canine hip. Vet Rec 1977;101:181–4.
19. Berzon JL, Howard PE, Covell SJ, et al. A retrospective study of the efficacy of femoral head and neck excisions in 94 dogs and cats. Vet Surg 1980;9:88–92.
20. Gendreau C, Cawley AJ. Excision of the femoral head and neck: the long-term results of 35 operations. J Am Anim Hosp Assoc 1977;13:605–8.
21. Lippincott CL. Improvement of excision arthroplasty of the femoral head and neck utilizing a biceps femoris muscle sling. J Am Anim Hosp Assoc 1981;17:668–72.
22. Lippincott CL. Excision arthroplasty of the femoral head and neck utilizing a biceps femoris muscle sling. Part two: the caudal pass. J Am Anim Hosp Assoc 1984;20:377–84.
23. Liska WD, Doyle N, Marcellin-Little DJ, et al. Total hip replacement in three cats: surgical technique, short-term outcome and comparison to femoral head ostectomy. Vet Comp Orthop Traumatol 2009;22(6):505–10.
24. Warnock JJ, Dyce J, Pooya H, et al. Retrospective analysis of canine miniature total hip prostheses. Vet Surg 2003;32(3):285–91.
25. Marino DJ, Ireifej SJ, Loughin CA. Micro total hip replacement in dogs and cats. Vet Surg 2012;41(1):121–9.
26. Liska WD. Micro total hip replacement for dogs and cats: surgical technique and outcomes. Vet Surg 2010;39(7):797–810.
27. Johnson KA. Piermattei's atlas of surgical approaches to the bones and joints of the dog and cat. 5th edition. St Louis (MO): Elsevier Saunders; 2013. p. 4–16, 322–35.
28. Evans HE, de Lahunta A. Miller's anatomy of the dog. 4th edition. St Louis (MO): Elsevier Saunders; 2012. p. 176–7, 254–67.
29. Mann FA, Tangner CH, Wagner-Mann C, et al. A comparison of standard femoral head and neck excision and femoral head and neck excision using a biceps femoris muscle flap in the dog. Vet Surg 1987;16(3):223–30.
30. Fitzpatrick N, Pratola L, Yeadon R, et al. Total hip replacement after failed femoral head and neck excision in two dogs and two cats. Vet Surg 2012 Jan;41(1):136–42.
31. Dueland R, Bartel DL, Antonson E. Force plate technique for canine gait analysis: preliminary report on total hip and excision arthroplasty [proceedings]. Bull Hosp Joint Dis 1977;38(1):35–6.
32. Anderson A. Treatment of hip dysplasia. J Small Anim Pract 2011;52(4):182–9.
33. Montgomery RD, Milton JL, Horne RD, et al. A retrospective comparison of three techniques for femoral head and neck excision in dogs. Vet Surg 1987;16(6):423–6.
34. Grisneaux E, Dupuis J, Pibarot P, et al. Effects of postoperative administration of ketoprofen or carprofen on short- and long-term results of femoral head and neck excision in dogs. J Am Vet Med Assoc 2003;223(7):1006–12.

35. Piek CJ, Hazewinkel HA, Wolvekamp WT, et al. Long-term follow-up of avascular necrosis of the femoral head in the dog. J Small Anim Pract 1996;37(1):12–8.

36. Yap FW, Dunn AL, Garcia-Fernandez PM, et al. Femoral head and neck excision in cats: medium- to long-term functional outcome in 18 cats. J Feline Med Surg 2015;17(8):704–10.

37. Prostredny JM, Toombs JP, VanSickle DC. Effect of two muscle sling techniques on early morbidity after femoral head and neck excision in dogs. Vet Surg 1991; 20(5):298–305.

38. Remedios AM, Clayton HM, Skuba E. Femoral head excision arthroplasty using the vascularised rectus femoris muscle sling. Vet Comp Orthop Traumatol 1994;7:82–7.

39. Dueland RT, Dogan S, Vanderby R. Biomechanical comparison of standard excisional hip arthroplasty and modified deep gluteal muscle transfer excisional arthroplasty. Vet Comp Orthop Traumatol 1997;10:95–100.

40. Tarvin G, Lippincott CL. Excision arthroplasty for treatment of canine hip dysplasia using the biceps femoris muscle sling: an evaluation of 92 cases. Semin Vet Med Surg (Small Anim) 1987;2(2):158–60.

41. Liska WD, Doyle ND, Schwartz Z. Successful revision of a femoral head ostectomy (complicated by postoperative sciatic neurapraxia) to a total hip replacement in a cat. Vet Comp Orthop Traumatol 2010;23(2):119–23.

BioMedtrix Total Hip Replacement Systems
An Overview

Teresa D. Schiller, DVM

KEYWORDS

- Cementless THR • BioMedtrix THR systems • Universal THR • Micro THR
- Nano THR • Collared BFX stem • Lateral bolt BFX stem

KEY POINTS

- Total hip replacement (THR) has become an accepted veterinary orthopedic procedure for treating a variety of coxofemoral joint disorders in companion animal patients.
- BioMedtrix, an industry leader in joint replacement, has developed THR systems to address the hip replacement needs of patients weighing from 2 kg to 80 kg.
- The most common complications associated with THR include luxations for both cemented and cementless THR procedures, aseptic loosening for cemented THR procedures, and femoral fissures and fractures for cementless THR procedures.
- Complications often require additional surgical procedures, but good patient outcomes and return of function is still achievable.
- A success rate of approximately 90% is a reasonable expectation for most THR procedures in small animal patients performed by experienced THR surgeons.

Total hip replacement (THR) has become a highly successful veterinary orthopedic procedure for canine and feline patients affected by various abnormalities of the coxofemoral joint. In 1990, the BioMedtrix company (Whippany, NJ) emerged onto the marketplace with release of its first THR implant system, the CFX (cemented fixation) system. The CFX system replaced the only commercially available canine THR system at that time, the Richards II system. The CFX system had implant modularity with 3 components: an acetabular cup, a femoral stem, and a femoral head. The cups and stems were available in different sizes but all matched a common femoral head size (17 mm diameter). The head attached to the femoral stem via a Morse taper fit. The 17 mm femoral heads were available as +0, +3, and +6 mm sizes to optimize femoral neck

Disclosure Statement: Dr T.D. Schiller is a Clinical Advisor and THR Workshop Instructor for BioMedtrix.

Clinical Programs, Department of Veterinary Clinical and Diagnostic Services, Faculty of Veterinary Medicine, University of Calgary, TRW 2D11, 3280 Hospital Drive Northwest, Calgary, Alberta T2N4Z6, Canada

E-mail address: tschille@ucalgary.ca

http://dx.doi.org/10.1016/j.cvsm.2017.03.005
0195-5616/17/Crown Copyright © 2017 Published by Elsevier Inc. All rights reserved.
vetsmall.theclinics.com

length to achieve appropriate joint tightness on hip reduction. The modularity of this system allowed better customization of implants to each patient. Improved surgical instrumentation was also developed, allowing a more precise THR surgical procedure. BioMedtrix has been an industry leader in veterinary joint replacement over the past 27 years. A variety of THR implant systems and designs, surgical instrumentation, and surgical instructional education programs have been developed to meet the changing needs of veterinary orthopedic surgeons and their THR patients. BioMedtrix manufactures THR implants and instrumentation for patients ranging in size from 2 kg to 80 kg. Implant designs and materials have changed over time in response to advancing clinical research and knowledge and surgeon needs in the area of veterinary THR procedures. The company estimates that approximately 28,650 CFX, 8900 BFX (biologic fixation), and 700 Micro THR and Nano THR procedures have been performed since the introduction of each implant system to the market place. This article is brief review of the BioMedtrix THR systems that are currently commercially available, the surgical procedure for their placement, and their associated complications and outcomes.

CEMENTED VERSUS CEMENTLESS IMPLANTS

Historically, THR implants relied on cement fixation using polymethylmethacrylate to achieve implant stability within the bone.[1–4] The 2004 Liska study of 730 consecutive CFX THRs provides the most comprehensive study data available describing this procedure, patient outcomes, and complications.[4] Collectively, these studies all reported high levels of procedure success and similar complications have been described, including dislocations, infections, femoral fractures, sciatic nerve neuropraxia, and aseptic implant loosening. The primary benefit of a cemented THR system is the immediate stabilization of the implants within the bone at the time of surgery. With resolution of their hip pain and hind limb dysfunction, patients are able to return to an active lifestyle with a relatively quick recovery period of 6 to 8 weeks. During the 1980s, aseptic implant loosening was identified as a significant issue in cemented THR patients.[2,5] Despite advancements in the surgical and cementing techniques of the THR procedure, the risk of aseptic loosening persisted.[6] Between 1986 and 1992, significant work in the area of cementless canine THR was carried out at the North Carolina State University College of Veterinary Medicine.[7–12] The Canine PCA (porous-coated anatomic) Total Hip System by Howmedica, Inc (Rutherford, NJ) was used very successfully for research and in clinical applications. This implant system was never made commercially available but data gained from its use resulted in the development and commercial release of the BioMedtrix BFX THR system in 2003. Cementless implants rely on osseointegration of patient bone into and or onto the implant surface.[13] Initial implant stabilization in these cementless systems is through press-fit. Precision acetabular reamers and femoral broaches are used for bone preparation. The implants are firmly and tightly seated into a prepared bone bed. The precise match of geometry and support by adjacent bone around the implant, combined with specific implant design features, works to maintain the implant position within the bone. A process similar to secondary bone healing is thought to occur with initial fibrous tissue ingrowth into the porous implant surfaces that then changes to bone ingrowth once a stable implant-tissue interface is achieved. Although initially less stable than a cemented implant, the biologic nature of cementless fixation has the potential benefits of a bone-implant interface that is stabilized by vital tissues with the potential for decreased risks of infection and aseptic loosening complications. In 2007, the BFX and CFX total hip systems were combined to form the Universal total hip system (**Fig. 1**). There was a standardization of the surgical approach and instrumentation for implant placement, and recognition that implants from both systems could be combined for hybrid THR procedures in which both cemented and cementless implants could be applied to a single patient for the best possible clinical outcome. No single THR system can meet the needs of every potential THR patient and having implant systems that work together with common surgical placement techniques benefits not only the surgeon providing these procedures but also the patients receiving them.

Implant selection for a THR patient will depend on a variety of factors, including surgeon experience and training, patient factors of size and body weight, disease process affecting the coxofemoral joint, bone quality, femoral morphology, and primary versus revision procedures. The application of cement in fixation of a THR implant can overcome some bone quality issues when present or in cases in which use of a cementless implant may be considered risky because conditions for initial press-fit cannot be achieved. Femoral stem subsidence describes a settling or distal migration of a cementless femoral stem postoperatively.[12] Femoral stem subsidence and rotational positional changes into retroversion can be a significant concern to a THR surgeon in the early postoperative patient while tissue integration into the porous surface of the stem is developing. Subsidence of a few millimeters is often insignificant to the patient but greater distances and significant rotational position changes may result in coxofemoral luxations, femoral fractures, and malaligned implants. Complex revision

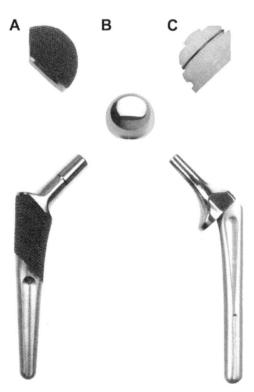

Fig. 1. BioMedtrix Universal THR Implants. Universal THR System consists of the BFX cementless cup and stem (*A*), a common femoral head (*B*), and the CFX cemented cup and stem (*C*). Multiple implant sizes are available to maximize for application in a variety of patient and bone sizes. (*Courtesy of* BioMedtrix, LLC, Whippany, NJ.)

procedures are often required to resolve these problems. Preoperative and operative decision-making regarding using cemented or cementless implants and surgical technique are key to avoiding these situations.

The Universal Total Hip Replacement System

The BioMedtrix Universal THR system includes BFX and CFX implants of various sizes that can be intermixed. A common surgical approach and technique for bone preparation and common surgical instrumentation have been developed for implant placement. Implant sites are initially prepared using the precise technique for placement of a press-fit BFX implant. If a decision is then made to use a CFX implant, minor modifications of the bone bed are required for a cemented acetabular component but the femoral canal will already be appropriately prepared to receive a cemented stem. This is a 3-component modular system, including an acetabular cup, a femoral stem, and a femoral head. A common femoral head will fit a BFX or CFX femoral stem and match a BFX or CFX acetabular component within a particular implant size category. **Table 1** illustrates the implant sizes and combinations available. The broad range of implants and ability for hybridization or combining both cementless and cemented implants provide significant implant flexibility and allows surgeons to choose what implants or combination of implants best meets the needs of their THR patient. **Table 2** lists the implant materials and manufacturing method.

Universal total hip replacement surgical procedure

Preoperatively, patients are radiographed with inclusion of a magnification marker placed at the level of the bone of interest. Knowledge of magnification and knowing

Table 1
BioMedtrix Universal total hip replacement implants

Stem		Head		Cup	
CFX	BFX	12 mm + 0	CFX	12 mm I.D.	BFX
#4: Maximum	#4: Maximum	12 mm + 3	18 mm		20 mm
patient weight	patient weight				22 mm
60 lb (27.3 kgs)	30 lb (13.6 kgs)				
CFX	BFX	13 mm + 1	CFX	13 mm I.D.	BFX
#4 or #5	#5	13 mm + 3	19 mm		20 mm
#4 stem/#5 neck	#6	13 mm + 5			
Maximum patient	#7	Additional 13 mm trial heads and cup			
weight 80 lb (36.4 kgs)	#8	impactors required			
#5	#9	14 mm + 1	20 mm	14 mm I.D.	22 mm
#6	#10	14 mm + 3			
#7	#11	14 mm + 5			
#8	#12	17 mm + 1	23 mm	17 mm I.D.	24 mm
#9		17 mm + 3	25 mm		26 mm
#10		17 mm + 6	27 mm		28 mm
		17 mm + 9	29 mm		30 mm
		17 mm + 13	31 mm		32 mm
		Special order			34 mm
		22 mm + 0		22 mm I.D.	30 mm
		22 mm + 3			32 mm
		22 mm + 6			34 mm
		Additional 22 mm trial heads and cup			
		impactors required			

Abbreviation: I.D., internal diameter.
Courtesy of BioMedtrix, LLC, Whippany, NJ.

Table 2
BioMedtrix total hip replacement implant materials, manufacturing method

Component	Material	Manufacturing Method	Implant Surface
BFX Femoral Stem	ASTM F136 grade 23 titanium Ti6Al4V ELI	Electron beam melting (EBM) machine taper, hand finish stem	NA
BFX Collared Femoral Stem	ASTM F136 grade 23 titanium TiBAl4V ELI	EBM machine taper, hand finish stem	NA
BFX Lateral Bolt Femoral Stem	ASTM F136 grade 23 titanium TiBAl4V ELI	EBM machine taper, hand finish stem	NA
BFX Lateral Bolt	ASTM F136 grade 23 titanium TiBAl4V ELI	Conventional machining from bar stock	NA
BFX Acetabular Cup Shell	ASTM F1472 Ti6Al4V ELI	EBM machined	NA
BFX Acetabular Cup Liner	ASTM F648 UHMWPE	Machined polyethylene	
CFX Femoral Stem	ASTMF75 cobalt-chrome	Cast cobalt-chrome Machine taper, hand finish stem	Bead blast Matte finish
CFX Acetabular Cup	ASTM F648 UHMWPE	Machined polyethylene	Radial and circumferential grooves
Universal THR Femoral Head	ASTM F799 wrought cobalt-chrome	Machined cobalt-chrome from wrought bar stock	
Micro THR and Nano THR Femoral Stem	ASTM F799 wrought cobalt-chrome	Machined cobalt-chrome	Bead blast Matte finish

Abbreviations: ASTM, American Society for Testing and Materials; ELI, extra low interstitials; NA, not applicable; Ti, Titanium; UHMWPE, ultra-high molecular weight polyethylene.
Courtesy of BioMedtrix, LLC, Whippany, NJ.

as accurately as possible the size of the bone to help choose the implant that appropriately fills the confines of the proximal femoral metaphysis and diaphysis, and the cranial to caudal width of the acetabulum, are key to successful implant selection and application. Although equally important in both cemented and cementless implants, the templating process for cementless implants is the start of surgical decision-making and planning. Four radiographic images of the pelvis and femur are taken preoperatively. A square ventrodorsal view of the pelvis with the magnification marker located at the level of the acetabulum is used for acetabular component templating. The standard lateral view of the pelvis is used to assess the shape of the pelvis and the relative dorsal position of the femur in relation to the acetabulum (**Fig. 2**A). A true representation of the femur is achieved by taking craniocaudal and open leg lateral views of the femur (see **Fig. 2**B). The magnification marker is positioned regionally at the proximal one-third of the femur in line with the level of the bone and it is essential that the length of the femur is parallel to the radiographic beam and plate. Implant sizing is carried out using calibrated acetate overlays or digital templates. Poorly positioned radiographs and inaccurately placed magnification markers can misrepresent the bone and may affect the surgical procedure and the incidence of operative and postoperative complications. Based on the work done with the Canine PCA cementless system, a femoral implant that fills approximately 85% of the femur is recommended to minimize the risk of implant subsidence postoperatively.[12] The appropriately sized acetabular component should match the cranial to caudal width of the acetabulum with the medial pole of the implant coming to or nearly to the medial acetabular wall.

At surgery, patients are positioned into lateral recumbency with superimposed hemipelvi in the sagittal plane. The patient is secured in this position through the use of a positioning device such as the BioMedtrix positioning board or a vacuum-assisted moldable bag. Stable and referential pelvic positioning is essential for accurate acetabular preparation and implant placement.

The operative procedure of the Universal THR system involves a modified craniolateral approach to the hip joint.[14] A femoral head and neck osteotomy is performed using a neck-cutting guide. The femur is positioned at 90° of external rotation and the neck-cutting guide positioned along the cranial aspect of the femoral neck, referencing off the long axis of the femur. Attention to the neck cut angle is important if placing a collared CFX femoral stem because the cut angle will dictate the alignment of the stem within the medullary canal when the collar contacts the bone edge during final implant seating. The final neck cut should be at least a few millimeters above the level of the lesser trochanter. Making a high neck cut that preserves cortical and cancellous bone proximally may contribute to better initial cementless femoral implant stability and torsional resistance while osseointegration is occurring.[15] Typically, the procedure then proceeds with acetabular reaming and implant placement; followed by femoral canal preparation and implant placement; a trial femoral head reduction to assess appropriate hip tightness and stability on reduction; and, finally, placement of the final metal femoral head with joint reduction and soft tissue closure. The same radiographic views of the pelvis and femur are repeated postoperatively to confirm implant positioning and evaluate the bone for any potential fissure lines or abnormal disruptions.

Surgical visualization and exposure of the acetabulum is established through the strategic use of Meyerding and Hohman retractors placed around the acetabular rim and on the proximal femur. The true acetabulum is identified through noting the location of the ventral transverse acetabular ligament. Reaming in this location is necessary to provide the most available bone stock for implant placement and achieving a stable interference fit between the bone and the BFX cup at its cranial

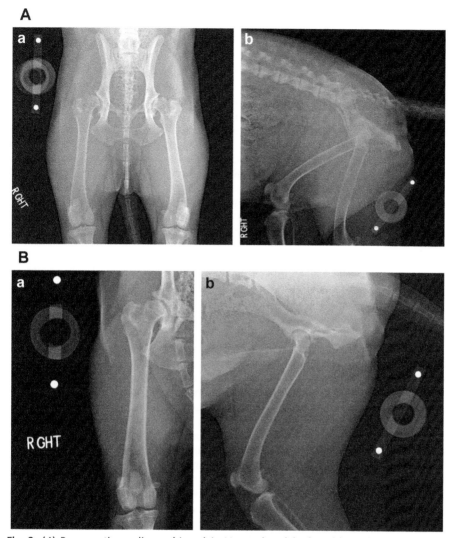

Fig. 2. (*A*) Preoperative radiographic pelvis. Ventrodorsal (VD) and lateral radiographs of the pelvis are obtained preoperatively. A 10 cm magnification marker is placed at the area of interest, parallel with the level of the bone for templating. The VD view (*a*) is used determine appropriate cup size. The walking lateral view (*b*) gives an indication of femoral head position relative to the acetabulum. (*B*) Preoperative radiographic femur images. Fully extended craniocaudal (*a*) and true open leg lateral (*b*) views of the femur are obtained to be able to accurately template the size of the femur. The magnification marker is placed at the level of the proximal one-third of the femur. Implant sizing is performed and evaluation of the central axis of the femur in both planes is determined.

and caudal poles. The ideal prepared bone bed, for optimal bone ingrowth, has exposure of healthy, bleeding cancellous bone cranially, dorsally, and caudally within the acetabulum.

Acetabular reaming is a 2-step process. A cheese grater–type starter reamer is initially used to remove subchondral and cancellous bone, and to achieve appropriate depth and approximate width of the preparation. The finishing reamer is a more robust, solid, and precise reamer. This reamer does not cut depth but simply finishes the prepared bed surface and width to within the 1 mm tolerance needed to allow press-fit of the particular size of BFX cup.

Specific attention to the process of reaming is key to meeting the goal of a placing a press-fit cup with proper anatomic axis. Instrumentation is used to ensure proper alignment and orientation relative to cup retroversion and closure angles. Reaming must be performed with minimal surgeon and reamer movement to ensure the precision in the size of the final bone bed. Ultimately, a prepared press-fit acetabular bed will be 1 mm smaller in diameter than the implant that will be placed within the bed. The BFX cup design is a hemisphere until the last 3 mm of the cup edge where it then becomes a cylinder. This change in shape is what provides the interference fit at the cranial and caudal poles of the implant that is achieved when the cup is seated to its full depth and becomes level with the adjacent bone edge. The metal-backed shell of the BFX cup provides additional support to the ultra-high molecular weight (UHMW) polyethylene liner and means less overall dorsal boney coverage is necessary to achieve adequate implant stability.[16] Needing less available pelvic bone for implant placement and the interference fit design makes the BFX cup very versatile and the preferred choice compared with a cemented CFX cup in almost all operative situations. When necessary, careful removal of the medial acetabular wall can be performed and a BFX cup can be medialized to ensure appropriate cup seating to engage the cranial and caudal cup poles level with the adjacent acetabular bone without risking the stability of the bone and pelvis.[17] The acetabular reamer for a particular size of BFX acetabular implant is used for trial sizing because the 2 have matching profiles for depth and width. Following final bone bed preparation, a trial CFX acetabular cup, 1 size smaller than the proposed BFX cup size, can be used to visually confirm desired cup position and confirm cup fit with the prepared bone bed. Using an impactor instrument and mallet, the cup is driven into the bone bed until final seating and depth are achieved. A significant benefit of the cementless BFX cup is that, if correct alignment and orientation are not initially achieved, minor position adjustments can be made or the cup can be completely removed and reinsertion performed again.

In rare situations in which a CFX cup is favored, the prepared acetabular bed is modified to create defects in the bone for cement intrusion and anchoring. Bone cement is cohesive, not adhesive. Three small key holes are created into the cancellous bone of the cranial, dorsal, and caudal aspects of the acetabular rim for cement movement into the bone to increase the shear strength at the bone to cement interface.[18] The bed is lavaged and dried as best as possible. Bone cement is mixed and placed with the bed and a CFX cup 1 to 2 sizes smaller than the corresponding size of the Universal finishing reamer is placed in the correct retroversion, inclination, and closure angles while cement hardening occurs.

The femoral canal is now prepared. A common surgical technique for either a BFX or CFX stem is used until the final implant choice is made. Ideal implant alignment matches the long axis of the femur in the cranial to caudal and medial to lateral planes. Entry into the femoral canal is achieved along the long axis of the femur through the trochanteric fossa, using an intramedullary pin. Sequentially, this opening is expanded using a drill bit, tapered power reamers, and increasing sized BFX femoral broaches until the final size of broach is reached to achieve the expected fit and fill based on the radiographic templating and the feel of adequate press-fit for a BFX stem. Each numbered broach correlates with a BFX stem size and the broach serves as the stem trial for sizing. The broaching technique must be precise. Broach alignment, in both planes, with advancement into the medullary canal creates the internal envelope and will dictate stem alignment and position. There is a significant learning curve for broaching technique and in recognizing adequate press-fit for the novice cementless THR surgeon. In general terms, with the final broach, the last 5 to 10 mm of broaching should be met with definite resistance to achieve final seating. This resistance is often coupled with a sound pitch change as the broach gets tighter within the bone. The femoral preparation for a cementless BFX stem relies on visual, auditory, and touch senses for assessing the adequacy of press-fit. It is during the final broaching procedure that the accuracy of radiographic templating is recognized. If excessive resistance is noted, one may be concerned that the broach is too large for the medullary canal or malaligned, and impending fracture or fissure of the bone could occur if broaching continues. Easy broaching or lack of resistance to broaching may be the result of underestimating the size of the bone or a general lack of cancellous bone quality and resistance to the broaching procedure. If resistance to broaching is lacking, this will not improve with placement of the implant. A decision to place a cementless stem where adequate press-fit has not been achieved risks significant postoperative complications associated with unscripted implant position changes. Femoral fissures, comminuted fractures, subsidence, and malalignment are common sequelae of inadequate realization of sufficient initial press-fit stabilization. The femoral stem is impacted to the desired depth within the femoral canal preparation with an impactor instrument and a mallet. The final resting position of the stem should be at the same level or within a few millimeters of the level of insertion into the femoral canal achieved with the final broach.

When press-fit cannot be achieved or patient factors dictate the use of a cemented implant, a cemented CFX stem is placed. CFX stem trials are available and are used before cementing in the actual femoral component. Trial stem placement is used to practice implant positioning within the femoral canal, to ensure the neck cut and the collar meet with the appropriate angle, to ensure axial placement of the implant within the femoral canal in both planes, and to check a trial reduction of the hip. This last procedure protects against cementing in a final implant only to discover that hip reduction cannot be accomplished and an adjustment of the height of the femoral neck cut was needed to shorten the femoral length and ease hip reduction tension. The femoral canal is flushed and suctioned to remove debris and fluids as much as possible before cement infusion into the canal. Placing a femoral cement restrictor is recommended for medium-sized and large-sized patients for implant sizes #5 to 12. This restrictor is made of polyethylene and is positioned at a specified level within the medullary using a specific measuring inserter device. The purpose of the restrictor is to keep the cement within the proximal regions of the femur and improve the ability for pressurization of the bone cement within the femoral canal, forcing it into the interdigitations of the cancellous bone and manufactured surface of the implant once it has been placed. The size of CFX femoral stem placed will typically be 1 to 2 sizes less than the final sized BFX broach used in canal preparation. This downsizing will allow at least a 2 to 4 mm cement mantle between the endosteal surface of the bone and the implant. In preparation for placing the CFX stem, a premade cement centralizer can be positioned over the tip of the stem. Care should be taken when handling the final stem. Studies have shown a greater than 80% decrease in the bonding strength between a stem and the cement if the stem is wet or contaminated with marrow or fat.[19] The stem centralizer has 1 mm wings that prevent direct contact between the metal stem edge and the cortical bone, and allow cement to encircle the tip of the stem between it and the edge of the cortical bone. Direct contact between the stem tip and the cortical bone has been suggested to predispose to cemented femoral implant aseptic loosening.[6]

Once the femoral and acetabular components are placed, trial femoral heads are used to assess the reduction tension of the hip joint. Optimal reduction should not be too tight or too loose. Also assessed during trial reduction is the match of femoral stem anteversion to acetabular retroversion, with the leg held in a neutral walking position, and identification of areas of potential impingement across the joint during range of motion. Failure to identify impingement intraoperatively, particularly on external rotation and adduction of the hip, could contribute to postoperative hip luxation issues. Lengthening the femoral neck through head size choice is carried out until appropriate tightness with full range of motion is achieved. The trial head is removed and replaced with a metal chrome-cobalt head. The surface of the final femoral head is highly polished to minimize surface defects that could result in abnormal wearing of the polyethylene cup surface. Care is taken to avoid contact of the newly placed femoral head during hip reduction with any metallic or abrasive surfaces to prevent creating accidental surface defects and scratches on it. Once final hip reduction and assessment are complete, the soft tissues of the surgical field are closed, in sequential layers. Postoperative radiographs are taken with attention to achieving the same position of the bones for implant evaluation as was achieved preoperatively.

A more extensive description of the Universal total hip surgical procedure has been reported.[20]

The postoperative care following a THR procedure involves limiting activities to controlled leash walks for 6 to 8 weeks, with a gradual return to full activity typically by 12 weeks. Patients are usually partially weightbearing on their operated limb within 24 to 48 hours of surgery and show a steady improvement in function over time. Body harnesses and belly slings are recommended to help provide rear limb stability during the initial few weeks of postoperative recovery. Acute changes in gait and weightbearing, especially during the first 2 to 3 weeks following a cementless THR procedure, often indicate a potential and sometimes significant complication and reassessment with radiographs should be performed. On successful full recovery, most THR patients will return to a full, normal active lifestyle with little to no limitations.

Universal total hip replacement complications and outcomes

The clinical outcome of cemented CFX THR procedures has been reported by several investigators.[4,21,22] Omstead's prospective case series of 51 cases had a complication rate of 7%.[21] Bergh reported retrospectively on 97 hips and reported a revision rate of 12.1% for the first side THR procedure.[22] Liska's 730 consecutive CFX THR procedures reported a successful outcome in 96% of cases.[4] The most commonly reported complications with cemented THRs are aseptic loosening and luxation. Less commonly, infection and femoral fracture complications can occur. Skurla and colleagues[23] reported on aseptic loosening in 38 THRs performed in 29 dogs. Postmortem evaluation was performed on these cases. Only 4 cases were found to have both stable acetabular and femoral components, whereas 14 dogs had loosening of both components. Femoral stem loosening occurred most commonly at the cement-implant interface. Edwards and colleagues[6] noted a similar site of loosening in 11 aseptically loose implants in 10 dogs. The mean time to aseptic loosening in these 10 patients was 30 months postoperatively. Postoperative luxation has been associated with several factors. Dyce and colleagues[24] suggest that cup orientation with an increased angle of lateral opening predisposes to dorsal luxation. Another study suggested that the angle of lateral opening and degree of cup retroversion were poor indicators of luxation risk.[25] Body type, size, breed, short femoral neck, and cup orientation were identified as risk factors for luxation by Nelson and colleagues.[26] Hayes and colleagues[27] identified that pre-existing hip subluxation or tissue laxity were significant contributing factors to postoperative hip luxation. Liska[28] reported a femoral fracture rate of 2.9% in 684 consecutive CFX THR cases.

Outcomes for the BFX cementless THR system have also been extensively studied. Roe and Marcellin-Little[29] reported on the short-term outcome of 204 cases performed over a 6 years. Forty-eight percent of patients had a zero complication rate. Minor complications that required no additional surgery occurred in 25% of patients. These included subsidence and stem rotation with and without associated fissures. Major complications occurred in 11% of patients, most commonly luxations (8.4%). Femoral fractures occurred in 4.4%. One case of sciatic neuropraxia was recorded. Two cups failed to achieve stable bone ingrowth and 1 was cultured positive for a *Staphylococcus* organism. No femoral stems showed lack of bone ingrowth. Return to normal weightbearing on the operated leg was noted by 3 months postoperatively in 35 BFX THR cases evaluated by Lascelles and colleagues[30] using a pressure-sensing walkway. Ganz and colleagues[31] reported on the risk factors for femoral fracture in cementless THR procedures. Older dogs and dogs with a lower canal flare index showed a higher risk of femoral fracture in cementless total hip arthroplasty procedures. In 219 BFX THR procedures performed in 183 dogs, a total complication rate of 31.1% was reported by Kidd and colleagues.[32] Catastrophic and major complications occurred in 17.8% of cases. Femoral fissures (46), femoral fractures (15), and coxofemoral luxation (9) were noted. Full return to function was achieved in 88.1% of cases with a median follow-up of 42 months.

Cementless BFX THR procedures have been successful but there is a learning curve. Case selection and adherence to precise surgical technique is important for minimizing fissure and fracture complications. These types of complications can decrease with experience. Roe and Marcellin-Little[29] noted a decline in their fissure rate from 30% in their first 50 patients to 4% in their last 50. Some surgeons have chosen to perform more hybrid procedures, opting for a cementless cup and a cemented stem to lessen the risk of femoral fissure complications. Gemmill and colleagues[33] reported on 78 hybrid THR procedures in 71 dogs. Major postoperative complications occurred in 5% (4) cases. Only 1 intraoperative femoral fissure was reported. The postoperative complications included 1 luxation, 1 femoral fracture, 1 implant fracture, and 1 case of aseptic femoral component loosening.

Micro and Nano Total Hip Replacement Systems

Functional restoration of a diseased hip joint through a THR procedure should be the goal for all potential patients, regardless of their size. Small dogs and cats are affected by pathologic conditions affecting the hip joint similar to those of larger patients. Avascular necrosis, degenerative osteoarthritis, femoral head and neck fractures, and coxofemoral subluxations and luxations create painful hip conditions and rear limb dysfunction for these smaller patients. In June 2005, the Micro THR system for small (<12 kg) canine breeds and cats was introduced. The Nano THR system followed in 2010. The Micro THR and Nano THR procedures allow restoration of normal hip biomechanics and function due to painful osteoarthritis and traumatic hip injuries in patients ranging in size from 2 kg to 12 kg.

The Micro THR system mimics the traditional BioMedtrix CFX THR system. It consists of the same 3-component modular system, an UHMW polyethylene cup, a tapered and collared femoral stem, and a femoral head (**Fig. 3**). As can be seen in **Table 3** there are different implant sizes to address different patient body weights, femoral and acetabular morphologies, and different sized femoral heads to match with different stems and cups.

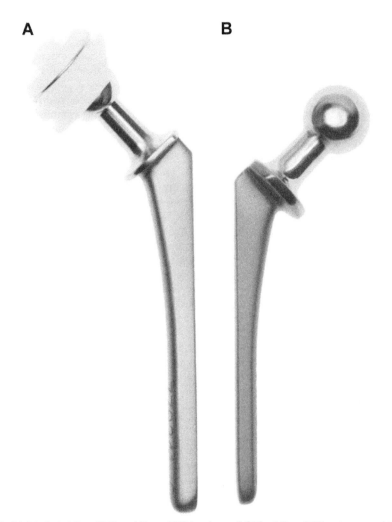

Fig. 3. BioMedtrix Micro THR and Nano THR implants. (*A*) The Micro THR system consists of a cemented cup, a modular femoral head, and a chrome-cobalt femoral stem. The surface of the stem is bead blasted to increase bonding of cement to the implant. (*B*) The Nano THR is a monoblock chrome-cobalt stem with a bead blasted surface. The 6 mm head fits with a 10 mm cemented cup (not shown) that is identical in design to the Micro THR and CFX cemented cups. (*Courtesy of* BioMedtrix, LLC, Whippany, NJ.)

The Nano THR system was developed for the smallest canine THR patients, in the 2 to 5 kg size range. This system uses a monoblock collared femoral stem with a 6 mm fixed femoral head (see **Fig. 3**) and a 10 mm UHMW polyethylene cup that is an identical but scaled down version of the traditional CFX cup. The femoral stem comes in 3 sizes reflecting different neck lengths +0 mm, +2 mm, and +4 mm.

The small size of these implants and the patients they are placed in necessitates that implants are stabilized by bone cement. The surgical approach to these patients is similar to that of larger THR patients. Templating of presurgical radiographs, taken in the same positions as for larger patients is performed to assess appropriate

Table 3
BioMedtrix Micro total hip replacement or Nano total hip replacement implants

	Stem	Head	Cup
Micro THR	CFX	8mm + 0	CFX 8 mm I.D.
	#2: Maximum patient weight	8mm + 2	12 mm
	#3: 40 lb (18.2 kg)		14 mm
			16 mm

	Stem	Cup
Nano THR	CFX	CFX 6 mm I.D.
	#1 + 0: 1 piece stem or head	10 mm
	#1 + 2: Maximum patient weight	
	#1 + 4: 20 lb (9.0 kg)	

Abbreviation: I.D., internal diameter.
Courtesy of BioMedtrix, LLC, Whippany, NJ.

implant sizing. The surgical preparation of the patient necessitates securing the patient in a positioning device to maintain pelvic alignment for proper implant placement and orientation. Specific instrumentation and trial implants have been developed and the procedure is largely performed similarly to a Universal THR procedure for placing cemented implants, with the primary exception that implant site preparations are done almost entirely through manual manipulations of surgical tools versus using power. Acetabular preparation is performed with solid fixed reamers on a shaft used in a Jacobs chuck. A high-speed burr can also aid in careful bone removal in acetabular site preparation. The femoral canal is opened using a small cutting awl and tapered reamer only under hand power to prevent accidental fracture of small femurs. A femoral canal cement restrictor is not used. Typically, the acetabulum is prepared, the cement mixed and delivered, and the acetabular component placed within the prepared bed. Attention to the same boney landmarks and matching the implant with the patient's acetabular axis and anatomy are as important as they are in larger patients for best outcome. Once prepared, the femoral canal is dried through suction. Cement is mixed and delivered into the femoral canal, achieving pressurization whenever possible and the femoral implant is positioned in axial alignment, in both planes within the femur. For a Micro THR, a modular femoral head is then chosen based on trial reduction and determining the correct tissue tightness across the joint. For a Nano THR, there are trial stems with fixed femoral heads of different lengths for use to determine the correct sized implant for cementing in place based on hip reduction tightness.

Reported outcomes of these miniaturized THR procedures has been reported as good to excellent in approximately 90% of patients.[34–36] The most commonly noted postoperative complications for the Micro THRs were coxofemoral luxation (9%–10%), femoral fractures (2% Marino), 1 case of sciatic neuropraxia, and 1 cup aseptic loosening.[34] The luxation and fracture complications in these studies were managed either through a revision or explantation procedure. In his case series, Liska[34] reported a 6% explantation rate and that no correlation was noted between luxation and angle of cup lateral opening. Undersizing and oversizing implants was the most common recognized cause of luxations. The most common complication reported for the Nano THR procedure was postoperative femoral fracture and this occurred in 3 out of 12 patients. One case of medial acetabular displacement occurred in this series of cases. Despite this 33% complication rate, all patients were thought to return to a good to excellent level of function by 12 weeks after surgery with either a revision procedure performed (fracture fixation) or a conservative therapy plan (cup displacement). All investigators comment that early technical surgical errors associated with the small size of these patients contributed to the postoperative complications that were noted. Increased surgeon experience and ongoing improvement of surgical instrumentation and techniques are expected to benefit the overall outcome of these types of THR cases.

Customized Cementless Femoral Stems

BioMedtrix has undertaken customization of the BFX femoral component to address unique patient presentations and surgeon desire to increase the overall level of confidence of implant stability in a newly placed cementless component. These customizations include a collared EBM (electron beam melting) titanium BFX stem (**Fig. 4**) and a Lateral Bolt EBM Titanium BFX stem (**Fig. 5**).

The additional of a collar or a lateral bolt to the traditional BFX femoral stem was driven by surgeon desire to provide additional protection against implant subsidence in the early postoperative and implant stabilization periods, especially in larger patients with more stove-pipe femoral morphology. Both implant designs have been used by multiple surgeons in multiple centers and have been shown to be successful. Minor modifications in the surgical technique are required for their use. During stem placement for a collared BFX stem, the final seated position of the stem is when the collar is within 2 to 3 mm of the osteotomy cut. It is expected that if a minor amount of implant subsidence occurs, the collar will come to rest on the bone and will prevent further movement of the implant distally into the medullary canal. It is essential to recognize that achieving adequate press-fit is still required for this stem to be successful. In the presence of insufficient resistance to broaching and implant impaction, suggesting inadequate press-fit, the mere presence of the collar will not guarantee against significant subsidence or implant rotation and the implant and collar can be driven distally through cancellous bone into the medullary canal of the femur. The collar should be oriented over the cortical bone to be most effective at preventing minor subsidence. Liska and Doyle[37] reported good results on the use of this stem with no significant subsidence issues in 110 consecutive cases.

The lateral bolt BFX stem brings in a fourth component to the modular Universal THR system. This system has just recently been made commercially available. The stem has been modified to allow placement of a screw-in straight bolt that is placed from the lateral cortex of the femur into the lateral aspect of the stem. The femoral component is placed using standard Universal THR techniques and is inserted to the desired level in the bone. A trial reduction of the hip is performed to confirm that hip reduction is appropriate for the level of the stem before preparing the bone to receive a lateral bolt. A drill bit and then a guide pin are oriented through a central canal in the femoral neck and body of the stem. The drill bit and pin are driven under power to exit on the lateral aspect of the femur, distal to the greater trochanter. A cannulated drill bit is then used to create a bone tunnel from the lateral femoral cortex toward the stem edge and the insertion site for the bolt. A depth gauge is used to measure the length of bolt necessary to fill the distance between the lateral cortex of the femur and the lateral edge of the femoral stem. An additional 2 to 3 mm of length is added to this measurement in choosing the size of the bolt to place. The bolt is inserted and screws tightly into the femoral stem. The bolt provides an additional locking mechanism for the stem and protects against both stem subsidence and rotation. Adequate bone quality and achieving acceptable press-fit stability are still required for this implant to be successful. Surgeons using the lateral bolt have expressed

A

B

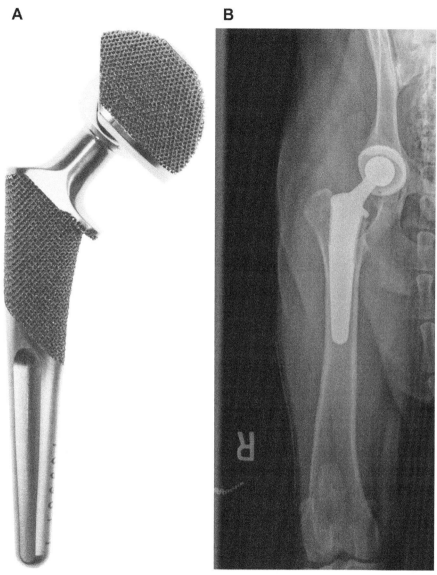

Fig. 4. BioMedtrix collared BFX stem and cup. (*A*) The collared BFX EBM titanium stem has a collar extended from the cranial aspect of the implant. The underside of this collar is porous to allow bone ingrowth. The collar is positioned at or just above the cortical bone edge of the neck cut and functions to potentially decrease the risk of subsidence. (*B*) A 3-month postoperative radiograph of a BFX collared stem in a 45 kg, 3-year-old German Shepherd dog. (Implant image Courtesy of BioMedtrix, LLC, Whippany, NJ.)

high satisfaction with it. This stem design allows a safer use of cementless femoral stems in larger weight patients and in patients with stove-pipe femoral morphology in which less matching of implant to bone geometry occurs when a cementless stem is placed, and in which the risk of implant movement is more concerning early in patient recovery.

A   B   C

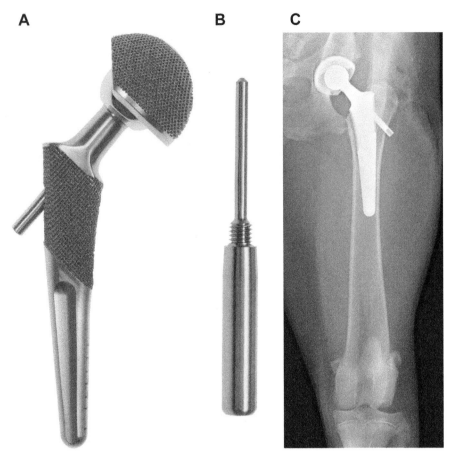

Fig. 5. BioMedtrix Lateral bolt BFX stem and bolt. (*A*) The lateral bolt BFX EBM titanium stem uses (*B*) a screw-in titanium bolt to provide an additional anchor point of the implant through the lateral cortical wall of the femur. (*C*) A radiograph of a 1-year-old, 42 kg hound mix taken 3 months postoperatively. (Implant images Courtesy of BioMedtrix, LLC, Whippany, NJ.)

SUMMARY

Within the BioMedtrix total hip systems there are many implant combinations that can be used to address a variety of patient presentations. Overall, cemented, cementless, or hybrid THR procedures can be very successful. Surgeon experience and adherence to the surgical principles of each THR system are key to surgical outcome. No single system is perfect or without the risk of some complications. Complications are usually manageable and it is reasonable to expect that most THR patients will achieve a satisfactory or better outcome with surgery. Future clinical and basic research will no doubt drive improvements in biomaterials, surgical technique, and revision THR procedures, providing patients with even better outcomes.

REFERENCES

1. Hoefle WD. A surgical procedure prosthetic total hip replacement in the dog. J Am Anim Hosp Assoc 1974;10:269–76.

2. Olmstead ML, Hohn RB, Turner TM. A five-year study of 221 total hip replacements in the dog. J Am Vet Med Assoc 1983;183:191–4.

3. Olmstead ML. Canine cementless total hip replacements: state of the art. J Small Anim Pract 1995;36:395–9.

4. Liska WD. Cemented total hip replacement: experience in USA with the BioMedtrix prosthesis. In: Proceedings of the pre-congress of the European Society of Veterinary Orthopaedics and Traumatology. Munich (Germany): European Society of Veterinary Orthopedics and Traumatology; 2004. p. 15.

5. Lewis RH, Jones JP. A clinical study of canine total hip arthroplasty. Vet Surg 1980;9:20–3.

6. Edwards MR, Egger EL, Schwarz PD. Aseptic loosening of the femoral implant after cemented total hip arthroplasty in dogs: 11 cases in 10 dogs (1991-1995). J Am Vet Med Assoc 1997;211:580–6.

7. DeYoung DJ, Schiller RA. Radiographic criteria for evaluation of uncemented total hip replacement in dogs. Vet Surg 1992;21:88–98.

8. DeYoung DJ, DeYoung BA, Aberman HA, et al. Implantation of an uncemented total hip prosthesis. Technique and initial results of 100 arthroplasties. Vet Surg 1992;21:168–77.

9. DeYoung DJ, Schiller RA, DeYoung BA. Radiographic assessment of a canine uncemented porous-coated anatomic total hip prosthesis. Vet Surg 1993;22: 473–81.

10. Marcellin-Little DJ, DeYoung BA, Doyens DH, et al. Canine uncemented porous-coated anatomic total hip arthroplasty: results of a long-term prospective evaluation of 50 consecutive cases. Vet Surg 1999;28:10–20.

11. Schiller TD, DeYoung DJ, Schiller RA, et al. Quantitative ingrowth analysis of a porous-coated acetabular component in a canine model. Vet Surg 1993;22: 276–80.

12. Rashmir-Raven AM, DeYoung DJ, Abrams CF, et al. Subsidence of an uncemented canine femoral stem. Vet Surg 1992;21:327–31.

13. Khanuja HS, Vakil JJ, Goddard MS, et al. Cementless femoral fixation in total hip arthroplasty. J Bone Joint Surg Am 2011;93:500–9.

14. Piermattei DJ, Johnson KA. Approach to the craniodorsal aspect of the hip joint through a craniolateral incision. In: Piermattei D, Johnson K, editors. An atlas of surgical approaches to the bones and joints of the dog and cat. 4th edition. Philadephia: WB Saunders; 2004. p. 290–5.

15. Townsend KL, Kowaleski MP, Johnson KA. Initial stability and femoral strain pattern during axial loading of canine cementless femoral prostheses: effect of resection level and implant size. Scientific Abstracts Proceedings of the Veterinary Symposium, Chicago 2006, American College of Veterinary Surgeons. Vet Surg 2007;36:E26.

16. Montgomery ML, Kim SE, Dyce J, et al. The effect of dorsal rim loss on the initial stability of the BioMedtrix cementless acetabular cup. BMC Vet Res 2015;11:68.

17. Margalit KA, Hyashi K, Jackson J, et al. Biomechanical evaluation of acetabular cup implantation in cementless total hip arthroplasty. Vet Surg 2010;39:818–23.

18. MacDonald W, Swarts E, Beaver R. Penetration and shear strength of cement-bone interfaces in vivo. Clin Orthop Relat Res 1993;286:283–8.

19. Stone MH, Wilkinson R, Stother IG. Some factors affecting the strength of the cement-metal interface. J Bone Joint Surg Br 1989;71:217–21.

20. Peck JN, Liska WD, DeYoung DJ, et al. Clinical application of total hip replacement. In: Peck JN, Marcellin-Little DJ, editors. Advances in small animal total joint replacement. 1st edition. Hobeken (NJ): Wiley-Blackwell; 2013. p. 69–107.

21. Olmstead ML. The canine cemented modular total hip prosthesis. J Am Anim Hosp Assoc 1995;31:109–24.
22. Bergh MS, Gilley RS, Shofer FS, et al. Complications and radiographic findings following cemented total hip replacement: a retrospective evaluation of 97 dogs. Vet Comp Orthop Traumatol 2006;19:172–9.
23. Skurla CP, Pluhar GE, Frankel DJ, et al. Assessing the dog as a model for human total hip replacement. Analysis of 38 canine cemented femoral components retrieved at post-mortem. J Bone Joint Surg Br 2005;87:120–7.
24. Dyce J, Wisner ER, Wang Q, et al. Evaluation of risk factors for luxation after total hip replacement in dogs. Vet Surg 2000;29:524–32.
25. Cross AR, Newell SM, Chambers JN, et al. Acetabular component orientation as an indicator of implant luxation in cemented total hip arthroplasty. Vet Surg 2000; 29:517–23.
26. Nelson LL, Dyce J, Shott S. Risk factors for ventral luxation in canine total hip replacement. Vet Surg 2007;36:644–53.
27. Hayes GM, Ramirez J, Langley Hobbs SJ. Does the degree of preoperative subluxation or soft tissue tension affect the incidence of postoperative luxation in dogs after total hip replacement? Vet Surg 2011;40:6–13.
28. Liska WD. Femur fractures associated with canine total hip replacement. Vet Surg 2004;33:164–72.
29. Roe S, Marcellin-Little D, Lascelles D. Short-term outcome of uncemented THR. In: Proceedings of the 2010 American College of Veterinary Surgeons, Veterinary Symposium. Germantown (MD): American College of Veterinary Surgeons; 2010.
30. Lascelles BD, Friere M, Roe SC, et al. Evaluation of functional outcome after BFX total hip replacement using a pressure sensitive walkway. Vet Surg 2010;39:71–7.
31. Ganz SM, Jackson J, VanEnkevort B. Risk factors for femoral fracture after canine press-fit cementless total hip arthroplasty. Vet Surg 2010;39:688–95.
32. Kidd SW, Preston CA, Moore GE. Complications of porous-coated press-fit cementless total hip replacement in dogs. Vet Comp Orthop Traumatol 2016;29: 402–8.
33. Gemmill TJ, Pink J, Renwick A, et al. Hybrid cemented/cementless total hip replacement in dogs: seventy-eight consecutive joint replacements. Vet Surg 2011;40:621–30.
34. Liska WD. Micro total hip replacement for dogs and cats: surgical technique and outcomes. Vet Surg 2010;39:797–810.
35. Marino D, Ireifej SJ, Loughin CA. Micro total hip replacement in dogs and cats. Vet Surg 2012;41:121–9.
36. Ireifej S, Marino D, Loughin CA. Nano total hip replacement in 12 dogs. Vet Surg 2012;41:130–5.
37. Liska WD, Doyle ND. Use of an electron beam melting manufactured titanium collared cementless femoral stem to resist subsidence after canine total hip replacement. Vet Surg 2015;44(7):883–94.

Zurich Cementless Total Hip Replacement

David Hummel, DVM

KEYWORDS

- Total hip replacement • Hip dysplasia • Cementless • Dog • Zurich

KEY POINTS

- Total hip replacement (THR) is considered the gold standard for treatment of intractable pain from hip dysplasia.
- THR procedures are divided into 2 main categories: cemented and cementless, with hybrid a combination of the 2.
- The Zurich Cementless THR system is a purely cementless system, which uses a combination of press-fit (acetabular component) and locking screw (femoral component) fixation.
- The Zurich THR system was designed to address the main challenge facing cemented systems (aseptic loosening) while providing the benefit of immediate stability with its novel locking screw implantation system for the femoral stem rather than a conventional press fit design.
- The Zurich THR system is reported to have similar success rates to other THR systems and is an effective treatment option for various orthopedic conditions of the coxofemoral joint in medium to giant breed dogs.

INTRODUCTION

Canine THR is an accepted method for treatment of various painful orthopedic conditions affecting the coxofemoral joint. The goal of THR for dogs with hip dysplasia is to return a chronically lame patient whose discomfort is refractory to conservative management to near-normal or normal function.[1] THR involves the surgical replacement of the femoral head and acetabulum with manufactured implants. Canine hip dysplasia, traumatic coxofemoral luxation, femoral head and neck fractures, and failed femoral head and neck ostectomy (FHO) are among the most common indications for canine THR.[2–6] Current THR systems can be broadly categorized as cemented, cementless, or hybrid (combination of cemented and cementless implants). Cemented THR systems achieve both short-term and long-term stability with the use of polymethyl methacrylate as the interface between the implant and bone. Cementless THR systems

The author has nothing to disclose.
Department of Surgery, Skylos Sports Medicine, 10270 Baltimore National Pike, Ellicott City/Frederick, MD 21042, USA
E-mail address: dhummel@skylossportsmedicine.com

achieve short-term stability by various methods depending on the implant system used (press-fit, locking screw fixation, or screw-in implants) and long-term stability via bone in-growth (on-growth) into implants.[5–7]

The Zurich Cementless THR (Kyon, Zurich, Switzerland) was developed at the University of Zurich in the late 1990s[6] (**Fig. 1**). The Zurich THR system uses a novel locking screw implantation system for application, coupled with a unique microinterlock bone on-growth for long-term stability of the femoral component. The Zurich acetabular component uses an initial press-fit stabilization followed by long-term stabilization via bone in-growth through a porous design of the cup (multiple small holes for bone in-growth).[8,9] Numerous publications have reported the surgical technique and outcomes for the Zurich THR.[3,6,10]

INDICATIONS/CONTRAINDICATIONS

Zurich THR has been reported as a treatment modality for canine hip dysplasia, fractures of the femoral head and neck, chronic or nonreducible luxations, failure of various hip surgeries (triple pelvic osteotomy, FHO, dorsal acetabular rim arthroplasty, and toggle pin procedure), and revision of THR performed with an alternate system.[3,6,10,11] There are no reported contraindications specific to the Zurich THR (Vezzoni A, personal communication, 2016). General contraindications for THR should be considered with the Zurich THR (**Table 1**).

Signalment for reported clinical cases of Zurich THR is varied but currently limited to medium to giant breed dogs. Reported breeds include mixed breed dog, German shepherd dog, golden retriever, Labrador retriever, Newfoundland, Rottweiler, Bernese mountain dog, border collie, pit bull, Belgian shepherd, Doberman, Hovawart, Leonberger, flat-coated retriever, greater Swiss mountain dog, Irish setter, Magyar vizsla, and riesenschnauzer.[3,6,10] Reported patient age at the time of Zurich THR is also varied, with ages ranging from 4.5 months to 12.6 year old.[6,10] Zurich THR is well documented in intact male dogs, castrated male dogs, intact female dogs, and spayed female dogs.[3,6,10]

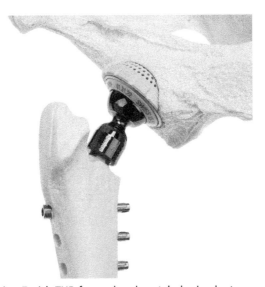

Fig. 1. Fifth-generation Zurich THR femoral and acetabular implants.

Table 1
Indications and contraindications for Zurich total hip replacement

Indications	Contraindications
Canine hip dysplasia	Infection
Fractures of the femoral head and neck	Neoplasia
Coxofemoral luxation (chronic or nonreducible)	Severe neurologic deficits
Failure of triple pelvic osteotomy	Concurrent cranial cruciate ligament
Failure of FHO	disease
Failure of dorsal acetabular rim arthroplasty	
Failure of toggle pin stabilization	
Revision of THR by alternate system	

TECHNIQUE/PROCEDURE
Preparation

Preoperative

- Minimum database (serum chemistry, complete blood cell count, urinalysis, +/− urine or blood culture)
- Skin evaluation for pyoderma
- +/− Buccal mucosal bleeding time
- Radiographic examination (with calibration device)
  - Lateral view of pelvis
  - Ventrodorsal hip extended view
  - Ventrodorsal frog-leg view
  - Lateral view of femur
  - Oblique caudocranial lateral view of proximal femur
  - Lateral view of stifle (ruling out stifle effusion)
- Client preparation and confirmation of side to be operated
- Selection and procurement of appropriate implant sizes
  - Measured stem size, plus 1 size smaller
  - Measured acetabular cup size, plus 1 size smaller
  - Necessary bicortical screws
  - Full range of neck lengths in planned diameter

Perioperative

- Wide surgical clip (midline of back dorsally to midline of abdomen ventrally, last rib cranially to anus caudally, and distally to metatarsus)[12]
- Purse string of the anus
- Metatarsus and distal limb wrapped in waterproof barrier
- Hanging limb prep with antiseptic (various) and an alcohol-based solution
- Entire patient is draped out (leaving only operated limb exposed)
- Full (exposed) skin draping with adhesive drapes or drapes sutured to the edges of the skin incision
- Double-glove technique, changing gloves after draping and prior to each point an implant is handled
- Limited personnel in the operating room, limited talking to surgical communication, suction used on demand rather than in a continuous mode

Patient positioning

- Kyon patient positioning device (**Fig. 2**)[12]
- Lateral recumbency with hip to be operated up

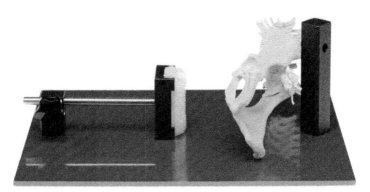

Fig. 2. Proprietary Kyon surgical positioner for operating table.

- Spine must be parallel to table with the bodies of the iluim superimposed
- +/− Fluoroscopy to ensure proper positioning of pelvis in a square and neutral plane

Approach

Surgeon is positioned at ventral side of the patient[12]

- Skin
  - Craniolateral approach to the hip[13]
  - 5-cm dorsal and cranial to the greater trochanter, extending down to midshaft of femur
- Fascia
  - Biceps fascia is incised and biceps is retracted caudally
  - Fascia lata is incised, preserving tensor fascia lata muscle
  - Fascial incision continued dorsally between tensor fascia lata and superficial gluteal
  - Lateral margin of deep gluteal tendon is separated from joint capsule and retracted
- Partial tenotomy of deep gluteal muscle insertion (tag deep gluteal tendon with suture, aiding in retraction and identification of tendon for closure)
- T-shaped or H-shaped incision in the joint capsule
  - Elevation of the cranial femoral insertion of the vastus lateralis muscle

TECHNIQUE/PROCEDURE
Femoral Ostectomy

1. Dislocate the femoral head and sever the ligament of the femoral head (using a Hatt spoon).[12]
2. Externally rotate the femur 90°. Assistant holds the limb in the position, with the stifle pressed toward the table and the patella oriented up.
3. Place Hohmann retractor under proximal femur to elevate to a horizontal position.
4. Using a single-action rongeur, remove the ridge of bone between the greater trochanter and the femoral head creating a groove (as lateral as possible).
5. Using an oscillating saw, perform the femoral head ostectomy:
   a. The ostectomy is straight, from the distal aspect of the groove (created in previous step) to just under the head and proximal to the lesser trochanter.
   b. The ostectomy is inclined approximately 5° to 10° to protect the capsular attachment at the caudal aspect of the neck (**Fig. 3**).

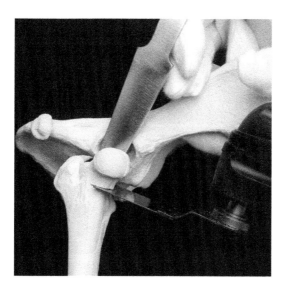

Fig. 3. FHO.

    c. While performing the ostectomy, cool the saw with a physiologic solution.
    d. The ostectomy should be visually checked to ensure the cut is parallel to the base of the neck of the stem implant.
6. Remove femoral head and save.

Femur Preparation

Surgeon assumes new position on dorsal side of patient

Reaming — initial preparation of femoral canal

1. If required to achieve a coaxial approach, the Hohmann retractor is repositioned more distally under the proximal femur.
2. Attach the primary reamer to the T-handle (according to size of stem to be used, **Table 2**).
3. Insert canal reamer into endosteal cavity, starting at the caudolateral aspect of the ostectomy (close to the origin of the external rotators of the hip), ensuring axial access to the medullary canal (**Fig. 4**).
4. Enlarge the femoral canal access by hand with half-rotations forward and backward. Start in a medial to lateral orientation, then progress to a more lateral coaxial orientation with the femur, aiming for the patella. Avoid excessive force when inserting or turning the reamer.

Table 2
Reamer and broach size for Zurich total hip replacement implantation of femoral stem

Stem Size	X-Small	Small	Medium	Large
Primary reamer	4.5 mm	4.5 mm	6.0 mm	6.0 mm
Secondary reamer	6.0 mm	6.0 mm		
Final reamer	8.2 mm	8.2 mm	8.2 mm	8.2 mm
Broach		3/4 length of small	Full length of small	Large

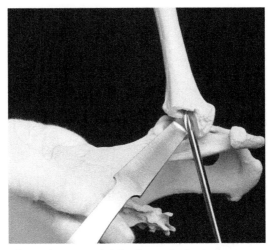

Fig. 4. Initial femoral reaming at caudolateral aspect of ostectomy.

5. Inspect and enlarge the canal with a rasp.
6. Remove osteophytes from the caudal margin of the trochanteric fossa with single action rongeurs.
7. Attach secondary/final reamer (see **Table 2**).
8. Rasp the femoral canal as needed between sizes of reamer. Rasp the medial aspect very gently, following the inner curve of the femur. Again enlarge canal access by hand with half-rotations forward and backward, aiming for the patella. Only the fluted portion of both the 6.0-mm and 8.2-mm reamers is inserted to avoid disruption of the distal endosteal vessels and to reduce the risk of vascular infarcts.
9. Enlarge the lateral aspect of the canal using the convex side of a Putti rasp. Collect the cancellous bone harvested by rasping; save for later use.

Broaching — final preparation of femoral canal

1. With the appropriately sized broach (see **Table 2**), use up and down strokes, without rotation. The broach is intended to remove bone laterally, so the smooth rounded surface of the broach should face medially. Rotation of the broach inside the canal can result in femoral fissure (**Fig. 5**).
2. Using the small fluted file, create the required stem anteversion. Avoid going deeper than the end of the file so as to not disturb endosteal vessels.
3. Create the proper seating and orientation (anteversion) for the stem. With the femur externally rotated 90°, the handle of the fluted file should be approximately 25° tilted cranially (not horizontal to the table).
4. Test the prepared femoral canal with the trial stem. Adjust the preparation of the canal until there is play in a few degrees of anteversion (approximately 25°).

Acetabulum Preparation

Surgeon returns to ventral position of the patient

1. Leg is repositioned in a neutral position. Gluteal muscles are retracted dorsally and the femur is retracted caudally.
2. A narrow Hohmann retractor is inserted and anchored caudally and ventrally to the acetabular rim.

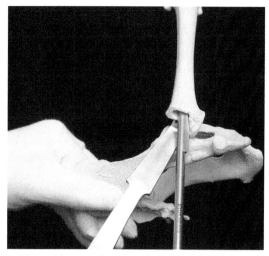

Fig. 5. Femoral broaching with smooth surface facing medial direction.

3. Enlarge the capsular incision and retract with Gelpi retractors.
4. Remove soft tissues from the acetabular cavity with a scalpel. Clear the remnants of the round ligament with rongeurs.
5. Palpate and preserve the ventral transverse ligament, which defines the ventral landmark for the position of the cup.
6. If the fossa is easily identified: using a reamer 1 to 2 sizes smaller than the final cup reamer, ream in the direction of the fossa (reamer shaft is oriented at 45° in the dorsal direction). Use a gentle precession of its axis toward 45° of inclination. Preserve cranial and caudal margins of the acetabulum, because they are required for proper press-fit of acetabular cup (**Fig. 6**).
7. If the fossa is not easily detected: the rough fibrocartilage surface ventral to the smooth eburnated surface provides a guide for the primary acetabulum. A pilot hole (2.5-mm drill bit in a medial orientation to the supposed fossa) can be used to gauge the depth to control the progression during reaming. Avoid reaming at 45° in the dorsal direction before identification of the fossa, because this compromises dorsal bone support for the cup.

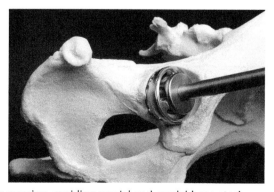

Fig. 6. Acetabular reaming, avoiding cranial and caudal bone stock.

8. Check subchondral bone consistency and preserve 2 mm to 3 mm from medial acetabular wall and a 1-mm to 2-mm step into the fossa.
9. Clean the fossa, removing all soft tissue remnants.
10. Using the reamer for the final cup size, proceed at low speed, in a medial and then dorsomedial direction, to 1 mm to 2 mm from the medial acetabular wall. Avoid reaming in the cranial and caudal direction, preserving this bone for the press-fit of the acetabular cup.
11. Using the T-handle, a final hand reaming of the acetabulum is performed to remove the rim of bone that is left after power reaming.
12. Perform osteostixis, using the 2.5-mm drill bit with drill sleeve and drill stop set to 3 mm. Drill as many holes as needed (based on size of patient) in the cortical bone of the medial wall.
13. Remove any osteophytes or soft tissue remnants found along the boney edges of the acetabulum. These tissues interfere with proper engagement of prosthesis to bone.

Stem Preparation

1. Change outer pair of gloves.
2. Collect 3 mL to 5 mL of patient blood from saphenous vein of the operated leg; add a few drops of tranexamic acid to syringe to promote clot formation.
3. Screw the stem into the jig, keeping it aligned with the 4.5-mm drill guide inserted in the most distal hole of the corresponding stem. Check alignment of the distal stem hole and ensure holding screw is firmly inserted. A poorly aligned or loose stem will make insertion of medial cortex screws impossible.
4. Place cup and stem implants into blood clot tray and pour in blood from syringe.

Fixation of Cup

Change outer pair of gloves.

1. Attach the appropriate size flat shoulder impactor to the impactor shaft (**Table 3**).
2. Insert the first orientation pin into the middle (45°) hole of the impactor shaft. Keeping this pin horizontal achieves a 45° angle of lateral opening.
3. Insert the second orientation pin into either the top hole (right limb) or bottom hole (left limb).
4. Check the patient's position, ensuring true lateral position (fluoroscopy if available).
5. Check impaction orientation, 15° to 20° retroversion of the cup is the guideline. The cup should sit symmetrically within the acetabulum, with the same amount of bone cranial and caudal.
6. Pack acetabular fossa with cancellous graft previously extracted from excised femoral head and femoral canal rasping.

Table 3		
Impactor size and cup hole guide for Zurich total hip replacement		
Acetabular Cup Size	**Impactor Size**	**No. of Rows of Holes Exposed**
21.5 and 23.5	Small	1
23.5	Small	2
26.5	Medium	2–3
29.5	Large	3–4
32.5	Large	4

7. Using the orientation pins for positioning, impact the cup into the acetabulum, covering the prosthesis with bone, both cranially and caudally.
8. Visually check cup orientation. Switch impactor shoulder adapter with the impactor ball.
9. Place impactor ball into cup and raise the shaft laterally until the bar touches the polyethylene liner. ALO of 45° = bar touching liner for 16-mm ball and bar 2 mm to 3 mm away from liner for 19-mm ball.
10. Inspect for proper retroversion. Fully seat the cup with heavy hammer blows. The pitch of the sound changes when the cup is fully seated.
11. Check the exposed rows of cup holes dorsally for proper seating of cup (see **Table 3**) (**Fig. 7**).
12. Inspect and remove any osteophytes that may contact femoral neck implant.

Fixation of Stem

Change outer pair of gloves.

1. Estimate head-neck:
   a. Seat impactor ball and shaft into the cup and hold vertically.
   b. Pull the leg distally (minimal Gelpi retraction).
   c. Place acetabulum drill sleeve between impactor shaft and femoral ostectomy.
   d. Use the drill sleeve (1.5-cm diameter) to estimate the gap distance (head-neck length). 1.5 cm gap = small head-neck; 2.0 cm gap = medium head-neck. Check for adequate (relative to dog size) clearance between cup and ostectomy and adjust as needed.
2. Recheck alignment of stem within jig.
3. Re-establish proper position and exposure of femoral canal.
4. Flush and aspirate femoral canal
5. Insert stem into canal with appropriate anteversion (matching the retroversion of the cup) until the base of the peg is at the level of the ostectomy (**Fig. 8**).
6. Maintain proper position of the stem (against medial femoral wall) by pressing down on the jig.
7. Insert screws:
   a. Maintain drill guide against periosteum.
   b. Screw insertion order: 3-1-5-2-4 (1 denotes most proximal, 5 most distal).
   c. Drill a 4.5-mm access hole using conventional drill mode.
   d. Flush screw hole of stem using 3.0 mm drill sleeve.
   e. Seat 3.0-mm drill sleeve into stem hole.
   f. Drill medial cortex with 3.0-mm drill bit using conventional drill mode.

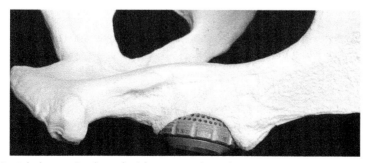

Fig. 7. Acetabular cup implanted with proper orientation.

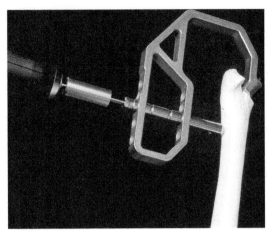

Fig. 8. Initial drilling with implanted femoral stem and proper position of jig.

    g. Insert screw until locked into stem.
    h. Place bicortical screw in the first stem hole (most proximal).
    i. Repeat steps for hole 5, then 2, then 4.
    j. Check and retighten all of the screws in same order as insertion.
    k. Remove jig using T-handle screwdriver

Reduction

Change outer pair of gloves.

1. Select head-neck. The position of the peg of stem can be used to estimate head-neck length.
    a. Peg touching dorsal rim of cup = short head-neck.
    b. Peg lying in center of cup = medium head-neck.
    c. Peg close to ventral border of cup = long head-neck.
2. Place head-neck on conical peg of stem.
3. Place femoral reposition hook around collar of head-neck, lightly hammer arm of hook to impact head-neck onto stem.
4. Pull reposition hook distally, cranially, and then medially, bringing head-neck over cranial aspect of cup to reduce the prosthetic.

Evaluation

1. Circumduction of hip joint should be free in all directions.
2. During abduction, ensure clearance between the greater trochanter and acetabular cup.
3. Pull test: pull head-neck with reposition hook distally and laterally; dislocation distance of 1 mm to 2 mm is acceptable.
4. Evaluate for risk of craniodorsal and caudoventral luxation.

Closure

1. Closure of joint capsule with interrupted absorbable suture material
2. Suture tenotomy of deep gluteal muscle with 2 rows of continuous absorbable suture material
3. Suture tensor fascia lata muscle to fascia lata with continuous absorbable suture material

4. Suture biceps fascia with continuous absorbable suture material
5. Standard subcutaneous and skin closure (nylon suture is preferred over staples for skin closure).
6. Sterile gauze is applied to wound and covered in adhesive bandage for 48 hours.

COMPLICATIONS AND MANAGEMENT

The documentation and management of complications after the Zurich THR have been reported in several large case series and case reports[3,6,10,14,15]; however, the follow-up and rate of complication differ depending on the published study (**Table 4**). Overall complication rate (perioperative and postoperative) for Zurich THR is reported from 16.4% to 26.3%.[3,6,10] Care must be taken when comparing these case series, because several variables are not consistent across all studies. In the case series from Guerrero and Montavon[3] and Vezzoni and colleagues,[6] all cases within each series were operated by a single surgeon with a high level of experience. In the case series reported by Hummel and colleagues,[10] cases were operated by 10 different surgeons with varying levels of experience. Mean follow-up for these case reports vary from 7 months to 48 months.[6,10] One case series[10] included perioperative fissure fractures and perioperative greater trochanter fractures in the overall complication rate; 2 did not,[3,6] making the overall complication rate reported by Hummel and colleagues[10] significantly higher. Guerrero and Montavon[3] reported 11 postoperative complications in 60 cases, all of which required revision surgery, with 1 case (luxation and subsequent infection) ultimately requiring explantation. Hummel and colleagues[10] reported 28 postoperative complications: 17 cases had various revision surgeries ranging from femoral fracture repair to explantation.

Certain intraoperative and postoperative complications may be more likely after specific technical errors. Over-reaming of the femoral canal can lead to intraoperative fissure fracture.[3] Prosthesis luxation is reported associated with several different technical errors, including inappropriate angle of lateral opening of the cup, inadequate anteversion of the stem, and inappropriate length of the head and neck unit.[3,10]

Table 4
Complications of Zurich total hip replacement as reported in large case series

Complication	Guerrero and colleagues[3]	Hummel and colleagues[10]	Vezzoni and colleagues[6]
Perioperative fissure fracture	1/60 (1.7%)	12/163 (7.4%)	
Perioperative fracture of greater trochanter		3/163 (1.8%)	
Postoperative femoral fracture	1/60 (1.7%)	3/163 (1.8%)	5/439 (1%)
Postoperative acetabular fracture		1/163 (0.6%)	
Transient neuropraxia		2/163 (1.2%)	
Prosthesis luxation	7/60 (11.7%)	12/163 (7.4%)	19/439 (4%)
Acetabular cup loosening (aseptic)	2/60 (3.3%)		9/439 (2%)
Stem loosening (aseptic)			4/439 (4%)
Implant failure	1/60 (1.7%)	4/163 (2.5%)	23/439 (5.2%)
Infection	1/60 (1.7%)	6/163 (3.7%)	3/439 (1%)
Cup, polyethylene wear			9/439 (2%)

The method of complication management is determined by severity, with some complications requiring minimal management (transient neuropraxia) and others requiring revision and/or explantation of prostheses. The most common indications for revision surgery include luxation, femoral fracture, infection, aseptic loosening, and implant failure.[3,6,10,14] The type of revision surgery performed depends on the nature of complication. Aseptic loosening (**Fig. 9**), luxation (**Fig. 10**), and implant failure (**Fig. 11**) can often be successfully revised with either adjustment to implants (ie, changing the angle of lateral opening of the cup) or replacement of implants with a different size (ie, increasing the length of the head-neck).[3,6,14] Fractures of the femoral diaphysis often require open reduction and internal fixation (plate and screw fixation)[6,10] (**Fig. 12**). Infections often require explantation, either temporary (Guerrero reported 1 case of explantation after infection, then implantation of new implants 2.5 months after initial explantation) or permanent[3] (**Fig. 13**). The reported rate of explantation after a major complication with the Zurich THR is 1% to 7%.[6,10]

It is accepted that postoperative periprosthetic fracture of the femoral diaphysis may be prevented with adjunctive fixation at the time of THR implantation. Adjunctive fixation with cerclage wire compared with lateral plating was recently investigated.[16] This study found that although both cerclage wire and lateral plating resulted in failure at higher loads compared with no adjunctive fixation, whereas only lateral plating resulted in a significantly increased peak torque at failure compared with controls.[16]

Several factors have been identified as increasing the risk of complication after Zurich THR. Increased preoperative body weight and increased preoperative and postoperative body condition score have been associated with an increase in the likelihood of complication.[6,10] Giant breed dogs are also reported to have a higher frequency of complications, namely implant loosening and luxation.[6] Older dogs with suspected significant bone fragility may have an increased risk of femoral fracture and, therefore, should have concurrent adjunctive femoral plating to prevent fracture (Vezzoni A, personal communication, 2016). Although patient age has not been shown to be a factor in the rate of complication, the types of complications encountered by young versus old dogs does seem different. Juvenile dogs seem more likely to experience acetabular cup wear or stem loosening, whereas older dogs are more likely to encounter femoral fracture, cup loosening, and cup fracture.[6]

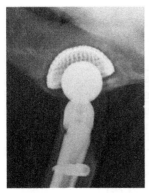 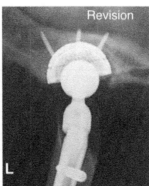 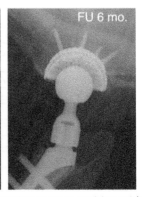

Fig. 9. German shepherd dog, 7 months old: aseptic cup loosening, 1-stage revision with special revision cup, and follow-up.

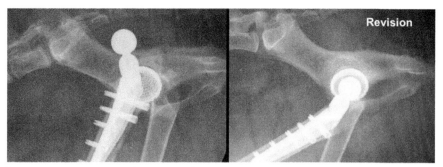

Fig. 10. Bernese mountain dog, 1 year old: dorsal prosthesis luxation 15 days after THR, revision with longer neck.

POSTOPERATIVE CARE

- Postoperative antibiotics for 5 days[12]
- Nonsteroidal anti-inflammatory drug therapy for 1 week to 2 weeks
- Skin suture removal at 10 days to 14 days
- Sedation recommended (as needed based on patient) for first 3 weeks to 5 weeks.
- Confinement in a safe, small, nonslippery environment for 8 weeks; leash walking only; no free-running, jumping, and playing.
- Clinical and radiographic re-evaluation at 8 weeks
- After appropriate re-evaluation, free activity is gradually re-introduced.

FOLLOW-UP

Most surgeons performing THR require extensive postoperative follow-up. A post-THR re-evaluation schedule of 2 months, 6 months, 12 months, and then yearly has been recommended.[6] Clinical re-evaluation of the postoperative THR patient should include evaluation of muscle mass, hip range of motion, gait analysis, and presence of pain on manipulation of the hip. Radiographic re-evaluation should be performed at each scheduled recheck and at any point where there is failure to meet expectations during the recovery. Radiographic projections should include a

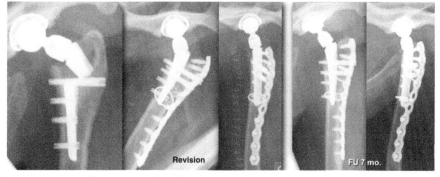

Fig. 11. Border collie, 7 years old, 26 kg: stem breakage 2.5 years after THR, with 7 months' follow-up.

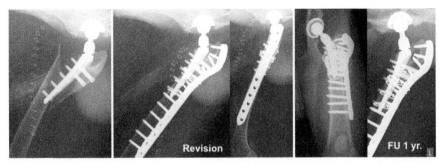

Fig. 12. German shepherd dog, 7 years old, 45 kg: femoral fracture 3 days after THR with repair and follow-up.

ventrodorsal view of the pelvis (**Fig. 14**), oblique projection of the pelvis (with the acetabular cup viewed fully laterally) (**Fig. 15**), and an oblique view of the femur (such that the x-ray beam is perpendicular to the screws of the stem) (**Fig. 16**).[6] Long-term follow-up of Zurich THR is highly recommended, because some complications are considered most likely to occur years after implantation (eg, stem loosening and polyethylene wear are reported to occur at a mean of 48–51 months after Zurich THR.[6])

OUTCOMES

Any outcome other than a normally functioning hip should be considered abnormal. Successful outcome after Zurich THR is highly influenced by postoperative complications. Although many complications can be revised with an excellent outcome, catastrophic complication (infection) often results in a poor outcome. Outcomes for Zurich THR are outlined in **Table 5**.

CURRENT CONTROVERSIES/FUTURE CONSIDERATIONS

There is some controversy in the use of THR for treatment of coxofemoral arthrosis in smaller breeds of dog and cats. This is largely based on the perceived success that these patients have with FHO surgery. In a recent systematic literature review on the surgical treatments for canine hip dysplasia, however, it was concluded that there is not sufficient evidence in the scientific literature to suggest FHO allows a consistent return to normal function for dogs with hip dysplasia.[17] The success of THR systems

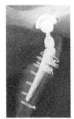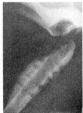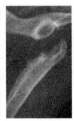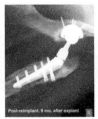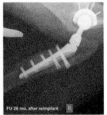

Fig. 13. Golden retriever, 1 year old: septic cup and stem loosening, explantation, followed by re-implantation at 9 months after explantation, with 26-month post-reimplantation follow-up.

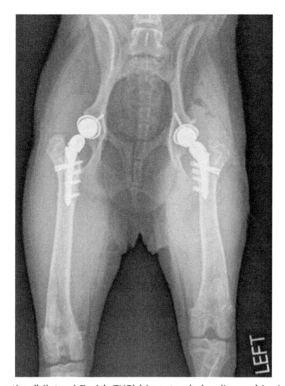

Fig. 14. Postoperative (bilateral Zurich THR) hip extended radiographic view.

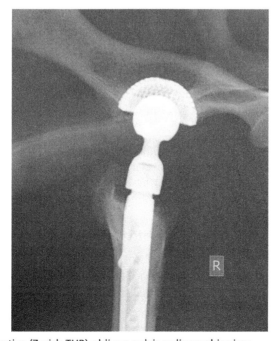

Fig. 15. Postoperative (Zurich THR) oblique pelvis radiographic view.

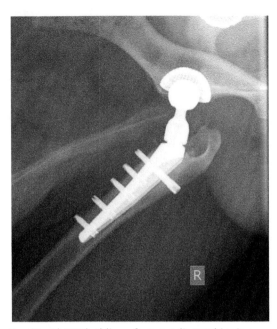

Fig. 16. Postoperative (Zurich THR) oblique femur radiographic view.

designed for small and toy breed dogs and cats has been previously reported for a different THR system.[18–20] Zurich has recently made available a mini Zurich THR system for use in small breed dogs weighing 10-kg to 16-kg body weight. Zurich has plans for the release of THR implants intended for patients smaller than 10-kg body weight in the near future.

Another current area of controversy is patient age/performing THR in young patients (<2 years of age). It is widely accepted that a majority of these young patients have excellent long-term outcomes.[5,6] Recent reports, however, have described cases of significant wear of the acetabular components as a long-term complication that was not previously recognized.[6,15] The cup wear and failure were 4 years to 5 years after THR implantation and may occur more frequently in large breed, younger, more active dogs or dogs with significant morbidity associated with the other limbs.[15] Several improvements have been made to the early generations of Zurich THR implants to combat cup wear, including the use of polyether ether ketone (PEEK) in place of the ultra–high-molecular-weight polyethylene and a proprietary wear-reducing geometry of the cup inlay (Vezzoni A, personal communication, 2016) **(Fig. 17)**.

Table 5
Reported complication rates and outcome for Zurich total hip replacement

Case Series Author	Overall Rate of Postoperative Complication (%)	Reported Successful Outcome (%)
Guerrero & Montavon,[3] 2009	17	97
Hummel et al,[10] 2010	17.2	88
Vezzoni et al,[6] 2015	16.4	99

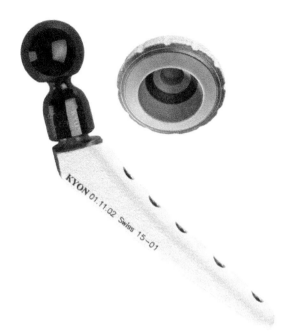

Fig. 17. Zurich THR implants with PEEK acetabular cup lining.

SUMMARY

The Zurich THR system has been shown to be an effective treatment option for various orthopedic conditions of the canine hip joint. Successful outcome is based on surgeon experience, a dedicated team of properly trained personnel, and proper case selection. Complication rates are similar to other THR systems and a majority of complications can be revised successfully.

REFERENCES

1. JKR. Surgical therapy of canine hip dysplasia. In: JSA, editor. Veterinary surgery: small animal. St Louis (MO): Elsevier Saunders; 2012. p. 849–64.
2. Schulz KS. Application of arthroplasty principles to canine cemented total hip replacement. Vet Surg 2000;29(6):578–93.
3. Guerrero TG, Montavon PM. Zurich cementless total hip replacement: retrospective evaluation of 2nd generation implants in 60 dogs. Vet Surg 2009;38(1):70–80.
4. Fitzpatrick N, Pratola L, Yeadon R, et al. Total hip replacement after failed femoral head and neck excision in two dogs and two cats. Vet Surg 2012;41(1):136–42.
5. Fitzpatrick N, Law AY, Bielecki M, et al. Cementless total hip replacement in 20 juveniles using BFX arthroplasty. Vet Surg 2014;43(6):715–25.
6. Vezzoni L, Vezzoni A, Boudrieau RJ. Long-term outcome of zurich cementless total hip arthroplasty in 439 cases. Vet Surg 2015;44(8):921–9.
7. Kim JY, Hayashi K, Garcia TC, et al. Biomechanical evaluation of screw-in femoral implant in cementless total hip system. Vet Surg 2012;41(1):94–102.
8. Bourne RB, Rorabeck CH, Burkart BC, et al. Ingrowth surfaces. Plasma spray coating to titanium alloy hip replacements. Clin Orthop Relat Res 1994;(298):37–46.
9. ST. Concepts of cementless Zurich prosthesis. in ESVOT 2004 Pre-congress Total Hip Replacement Seminar. Munich, 2004.

10. Hummel DW, Lanz OI, Werre SR. Complications of cementless total hip replacement. A retrospective study of 163 cases. Vet Comp Orthop Traumatol 2010; 23(6):424–32.

11. Andreoni AA, Guerrero TG, Hurter K, et al. Revision of an unstable HELICA endoprosthesis with a Zurich cementless total hip replacement. Vet Comp Orthop Traumatol 2010;23(3):177–81.

12. Vezzoni A. Zurich cementless total hip replacement surgical technique. Kyon Inc; 2014. 1.3.

13. Piermattei DL, Johnson KA. An atlas of surgical approaches to the bones and joints of dogs and cats. Philadelphia: W. B Saunders Comapny; 2004.

14. Vezzoni L, Montinaro V, Vezzoni A. Use of a revision cup for treatment of Zurich cementless acetabular cup loosening. Surgical technique and clinical application in 31 cases. Vet Comp Orthop Traumatol 2013;26(5):408–15.

15. Nesser VE, Kowaleski MP, Boudrieau RJ. Severe polyethylene wear requiring revision total hip arthroplasty in three dogs. Vet Surg 2016;45(5):664–71.

16. Pozzi A, Peck JN, Chao P, et al. Mechanical evaluation of adjunctive fixation for prevention of periprosthetic femur fracture with the Zurich cementless total hip prosthesis. Vet Surg 2013;42(5):529–34.

17. Bergh MS, Budsberg SC. A systematic review of the literature describing the efficacy of surgical treatments for canine hip dysplasia (1948-2012). Vet Surg 2014; 43(5):501–6.

18. Liska WD. Micro total hip replacement for dogs and cats: surgical technique and outcomes. Vet Surg 2010;39(7):797–810.

19. Ireifej S, Marino D, Loughin C. Nano total hip replacement in 12 dogs. Vet Surg 2012;41(1):130–5.

20. Marino DJ, Ireifej SJ, Loughin CA. Micro total hip replacement in dogs and cats. Vet Surg 2012;41(1):121–9.

INNOPLANT Total Hip Replacement System

Tisha A.M. Harper, DVM, MS, CCRP

KEYWORDS

- Total hip replacement • HELICA endoprosthesis • Cementless total hip system
- Screw-in endoprosthesis • Hip dysplasia • Coxofemoral osteoarthritis

KEY POINTS

- Total hip replacement (THR) is a salvage procedure that can be used to treat dogs with clinical signs of hip dysplasia refractory to any other treatment.
- THR can return a pet to normal or near-normal function after surgery.
- There is a potentially shorter learning curve using the INNOPLANT screw-in components and they may be easier to implant than other commercially available THR systems.
- Coxofemoral luxation has not been reported as a complication after implantation of screw-in THR components in dogs.
- Aseptic loosening is the most commonly reported complication after surgery using screw-in components in dogs.

INTRODUCTION

Hip dysplasia is a developmental orthopedic disease more commonly seen in large-breed and giant-breed dogs.[1,2] The disease is characterized by persistent laxity in the coxofemoral joint, which can eventually lead to coxofemoral osteoarthritis.[1,2] Hip dysplasia can be managed medically (conservatively) or surgically. Factors influencing which treatment is chosen include

- Age of the patient
- Severity of clinical signs
- Physical examination and radiographic findings
- Presence of other orthopedic diseases and other comorbidities
- Breed and temperament
- Expected patient performance
- Financial constraints of the client
- Skill of the surgeon
- Internal fixation devices available

Disclosure Statement: The author has nothing to disclose.
Department of Veterinary Clinical Medicine, University of Illinois College of Veterinary Medicine, 1008 West Hazelwood Drive, Urbana, IL 61802, USA
E-mail address: taharper@illinois.edu

Vet Clin Small Anim 47 (2017) 935–944
http://dx.doi.org/10.1016/j.cvsm.2017.03.003

THR is a salvage procedure that should be considered in patients with debilitating coxofemoral osteoarthritis secondary to trauma or hip dysplasia or that have failed conservative management for hip dysplasia. Other indications for THR include irreparable fractures of the acetabulum or femoral head, failed femoral head and neck excision, and traumatic coxofemoral luxation (acute or chronic).[3] Salvage procedures aim to preserve function in the limb and eliminate pain and should result in an improved quality of life. THR involves replacing the diseased femoral head and acetabulum with prosthetic components. Generally, THR systems are classified as cemented or cementless. The 2 more commonly known commercially available THR systems for small animal patients are the BioMedtrix Universal Total Hip Replacement system (BioMedtrix, Whippany, New Jersey), which has both cementless (biologic fixation [BFX]) and cemented (cement fixation [CFX]) implants, and the Zurich Cementless THR (Kyon, Zurich, Switzerland). Complications that have been reported after THR using the BioMedtrix and Zurich systems include sciatic neuropraxia, infection, septic and aseptic acetabular cup and femoral stem loosening, luxation, perioperative and postoperative femur fracture, wear of the polyethylene cup, and subsidence.[3,4] The INNOPLANT Total Hip Replacement system (INNO-PLANT Veterinary, Hannover, Germany) also has both cemented and cementless components (**Fig. 1**). Cemented (CemtA Cup) and cementless (Screw Cup) acetabular cups are available as well as 3 different femoral stem components, 2 cementless (HELICA TPS stem and 3Con Stem) and 1 cemented (CemtA Stem) (**Fig. 2**). Unique to the INNOPLANT Total Hip Replacement system, however, are the screw-in cementless femoral stem (HELICA TPS stem) and acetabular (Screw Cup) components (see **Fig. 1**). These components were developed to address some of the

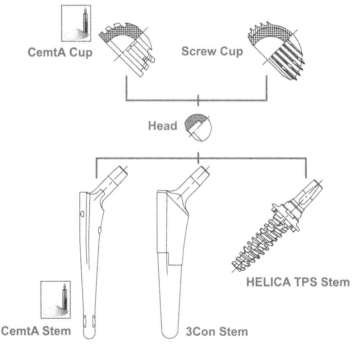

Fig. 1. Components of the INNOPLANT Total Hip Replacement system. Note the unique screw-in acetabular (Screw Cup) and femoral stem (HELICA TPS) components. (*Courtesy of* INNOPLANT Veterinary, Hannover, Germany.)

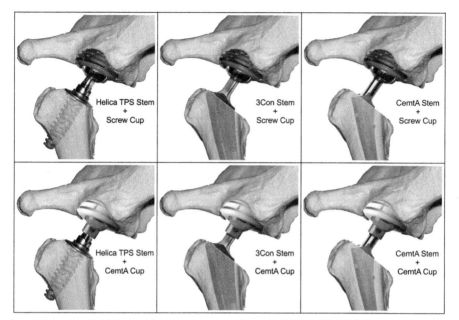

Fig. 2. Cemented and cementless components of the INNOPLANT Total Hip Replacement system. Note that both the cemented (CemtA Cup) and screw-in (Screw Cup) acetabular cups can be used with each of the femoral stems: cemented (CemtA Stem) and cementless (3Con-Stem; HELICA TPS stem). (*Courtesy of* INNOPLANT Veterinary, Hannover, Germany.)

concerns with the conventional THR systems, primarily to increase stability of the bone-implant interface to decrease micromotion and to decrease stress shielding of the bone.[5] The remainder of this discussion focuses on the unique screw-in components of the INNOPLANT Total Hip Replacement system. The screw-in components were formerly referred to as the HELICA Canine Cementless Hip System and have also been described as the HELICA-endoprosthesis in the veterinary literature. These terms both refer to the first generation of screw-in implants and will be used in this review as they were used in the past literature.

The materials used in manufacturing the acetabular and femoral screw-in components are similar to the other cementless systems[6]:

- The femoral stem and acetabular cup shell are made of machined titanium alloy. Initial stability is provided by the macro self-tapping threads present on both the femoral stem and acetabular cup shell that allow them to be screwed into prepared surfaces. This design allows for force-controlled implantation, which should allow for the implants to be firmly anchored in the bone.[7] The surfaces are rough-blasted to create a roughened surface that allows for bony ongrowth and osseointegration over time, thus providing long-term stability.[7]
- A flange is also present on the femoral stem (first generation) that seats against the femoral neck to improve stability and load transfer.
- The acetabular insert, which articulates directly with the femoral head, is made of high-density ultrahigh–molecular-weight polyethylene (**Fig. 3**).
- The femoral head is made of machined 316L stainless steel, which is then coated with titanium nitride to produce a very hard, wear-resistant bearing surface.[6]

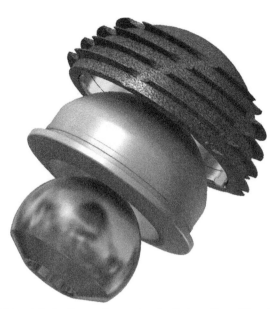

Fig. 3. INNOPLANT acetabular Screw Cup and polyethylene liner. (*Courtesy of* INNOPLANT Veterinary, Hannover, Germany.)

Potential advantages of using screw-in endoprostheses[5,8] are

1. Shorter surgery time that could decrease the chances of surgical site infection
2. Shorter learning curve
3. Less complicated revisions
4. Ease of implantation
5. Bone-sparing implantation because the stem is anchored in the metaphysis instead of the diaphysis; therefore, reaming of the femoral diaphysis is not necessary
6. Lower incidence of luxation due to greater tolerance for deviations from the normal angles of retroversion and ventroversion
7. Femoral neck anteversion is preserved because the femoral neck is maintained during the procedure, thus maintaining normal biomechanics of the joint.
8. The presence of the large positive profile threads provides an increased surface area and thus increased stability.

The eventual bony ongrowth/ingrowth for cementless implants is dependent on the initial stability of the implant.[9] The theory behind the increased stability of the screw-in system, based on studies evaluating the effect of compaction of bone in canine femora, is that during insertion of the femoral prosthesis the trabeculae are broken and compressed, resulting in increased peri-implant bone density and thus better anchoring of the femoral stem prosthesis.[9,10] Also, stress reduction at the bone-implant interface may occur due to an increased implant surface projected orthogonally to the direction of the force.[11]

INDICATIONS/CONTRAINDICATIONS

Indications for THR are nonseptic debilitating osteoarthritis, failed conservative management of hip dysplasia, failure of other surgical procedures to alleviate clinical signs associated with hip dysplasia, capital physeal fractures, traumatic coxofemoral luxation secondary to hip dysplasia, irreparable fractures of the femoral head and acetabulum, avascular necrosis of the femoral head, and failed femoral head and neck excision.[3,4] THR should not be performed in patients until there is closure of the acetabular growth plates. Generally THR is performed as late as possible in an animal's life; however, other factors that need to be taken into consideration include evaluation of muscle mass, weight shifting, and owner's impression of the success or failure of other treatments (medical or other surgical procedures) to maintain quality of life and function of the patient.[4,12] In immature patients with severe subluxation or luxation, consideration should be given to performing surgery earlier because morphologic changes, such as acetabular hypoplasia, dorsal acetabular rim wear, lateralization of the proximal femur, and muscle atrophy, can make later surgery more challenging.[12] Concurrent orthopedic disease, for example, cranial cruciate ligament rupture, should be addressed prior to THR.

Septic arthritis is an absolute contraindication for THR.[12] THR should not be performed if concurrent medical conditions, such as bacterial dermatitis, urinary tract infection, otitis externa, and severe dental disease, are present. These should be resolved prior to THR surgery. Significant client counseling is recommended and considered necessary when considering THR in patients with neoplasia; coagulopathy; compensated heart, liver, or renal failure; or immunosuppression, for example, diabetes, Cushing disease, and generalized immune-mediated polyarthropathy. Caution is needed when considering THR in these patients.[12]

TECHNIQUE

Templates are available (INNOPLANT Total Hip Replacement system) for preoperative planning. Standard preoperative and perioperative protocols are used. A standard craniolateral approach to the hip can be used to access the coxofemoral joint.[13] The details of the implantation procedure were originally described in the literature by Hach and Delfs.[8] The most significant difference between the preparation of the proximal femur for the screw-in endoprosthesis compared with the BioMedtrix and Zurich systems is that the osteotomy is performed at the junction of the femoral head and neck based on the prosthesis size, thus maintaining the femoral neck.[8] Also, the screw-in femoral prosthesis is implanted in the proximal femoral metaphysis and does not extend into the diaphysis; therefore, reaming of the femoral shaft is not performed.[8] After surgery, postoperative lateral and frog leg positioned radiographs are taken to assess correct prosthesis placement.

COMPLICATIONS AND MANAGEMENT

Complications reported with THR include coxofemoral luxation, infection, septic and aseptic implant loosening, implant subsidence, stem malpositioning, stem insertion complications, femoral cortex penetration, femoral fracture, sciatic neuropraxia, femoral medullary infarction, and pulmonary embolism.[14–21] Unlike the more commonly used conventional THR systems in dogs and cats, there are just a handful of reports in the veterinary literature documenting complications associated with the first-generation INNOPLANT Total Hip Replacement system screw-in components (HELICA Canine Cementless Hip System/HELICA-endoprosthesis).[8,22–25]

Hach and Delfs[8] reported on the initial use of the originally described HELICA-endoprosthesis in 40 dogs. Complications noted were resorption of bone under the segmented collar of the femoral prosthesis (2 cases), sciatic neuropraxia (1 case), femur fissure during implantation of the stem (1 case), femoral neck fracture (1 case), acetabular cup loosening (4 cases), and femoral prosthesis loosening (1 case). The investigators suggested that heat generated during the femoral osteotomy may have led to necrosis of bone and subsequent resorption of the femoral neck, or that stress-shielding, as seen in human prostheses, may have played a role.[8] Successful revision using a larger acetabular cup was achieved in 3 cases of acetabular cup loosening. In the case of the femoral neck fracture, excision arthroplasty was performed. Replacement of a loose femoral prosthesis was also performed successfully in 1 case. Most of the complications in this study were attributed to technical errors during the learning phase, and the investigators noted that revisions for acetabular cup loosening were relatively easy to perform. Other reports of complications after implantation of screw-in components include 1 case of septic acetabular cup loosening, which was successfully revised using a hybrid BioMedtrix BFX cementless acetabular cup and CFX cemented femoral stem[23]; 1 case of aseptic loosening of both components, which was successfully revised using the Zurich Cementless system[24]; and 1 case of a loose femoral prosthesis that was revised using a standard BioMedtrix BFX long stem cementless femoral prosthesis.[25] Aseptic loosening in 5 of 15 (33.3%) dogs within 1 year post-implantation of the first-generation screw-in components (HELICA-endoprosthesis) was seen in 1 study. The implants were removed in these cases.[22] To the author's knowledge there are no reports of coxofemoral luxation associated with the screw-in endoprostheses in the literature. In 1 study the investigators noted that there were significant deviations of retroversion and ventroversion of the acetabular cups; however, no luxations were noted. They suggested that correction for femoral neck anteversion was not necessary because the femoral neck was maintained. The originally described screw-in endoprostheses and surgical technique were used in that study.[8]

POSTOPERATIVE CARE

Postoperative care is similar to other THR systems but varies based on surgeon experience and preference:

- Appropriate analgesics
- Restricted activity to nonslip surfaces indoors for the first 6 to 8 weeks
- Activity limited to walking only outdoors on a leash for elimination purposes for a few minutes several times a day, with sling support if needed. No running, jumping, playing, stair climbing, or roughhousing with other pets is allowed during the first 6 weeks.
- Radiographs should be taken 1 month and 2 months to 3 months postsurgery
- Re-evaluate at 3 months, 6 months, and 1 year.
- Postoperative rehabilitation may be needed in select cases, for example, tight periarticular muscles after surgery that reduce range of motion.

OUTCOMES

There are no long-term studies evaluating outcome after implantation of screw-in endoprostheses for THR in dogs. The largest study (40 dogs) evaluating outcome noted that all patients were sent home by the second day after surgery. Follow-up radiographs were taken 6 weeks, 6 months, and 1 year after surgery.[8] Animals that had normal radiographic findings at their 6-week postsurgery evaluation were allowed to return to full mobility. In 36 cases, radiographic follow-up within 60 days revealed stable bony anchorage of the prosthesis components. Aseptic loosening, femur fissure, and femur fracture were complications noted in this study and most of the complications were seen within 6 months after surgery.[8] In a retrospective study of 16 dogs, 6 had loosening of the femoral stem by 1 year postimplantation.[22] One case had a positive intraoperative aerobic bacterial culture. The implants were removed in all 6 dogs. The investigators did not identify risk factors for loosening of the femoral stem.

CURRENT CONTROVERSIES/FUTURE CONSIDERATIONS

Despite the suggestions that less bone removal and more normal anatomic structure should retain the original biomechanics of the joint by maintaining proximal femoral load, an in vitro biomechanical study found that the first-generation screw-in femoral prosthesis (HELICA Canine Cementless Hip System) alters strain distribution in the proximal aspect of the femur and exhibits initial micromotion.[7] This may explain the aseptic loosening of the femoral stem seen after implantation and was thought a possible contributing factor in 1 study.[22] Loosening of the acetabular cup may also be an inciting factor for femoral stem loosening.[22] Hach and Delfs[8] and Andreoni and colleagues[24] also reported premature loosening of the first-generation screw-in endoprostheses. Kim and colleagues[7] also found that after implantation of the femoral prosthesis, strains decreased on the cranial, medial, and lateral cortical surfaces of the proximal diaphysis, with the caudal surface showing a significant increase in compressive strain possibly due to a significant increase in neck angle and subsequent load transfer through the tip of the implant. This stress shielding in the proximal diaphysis may be the cause of the bone resorption under the collar of the femoral implant seen in the study by Hach and Delfs.[8] The original screw-in femoral prosthesis was overall found to have limitations similar to other conventional femoral prostheses, that is, stress shielding and initial micromotion, but can withstand higher yield loads before failing in a similar mode as normal femora.[7] Concerns with initial implant instability and subsequent loosening have led to modifications in the technique for femoral prosthesis implantation, to enhance stability by engaging the lateral femoral cortex[5,26]:

- A shorter femoral neck, that is, more distal osteotomy, has been suggested to achieve lateralization of the femoral prosthesis and to engage the lateral femoral cortex. Although this may enhance stability, the proposed biomechanical benefit of maintaining the length of the original femoral neck to maintain version angles and angle of inclination of the original femoral neck are likely lost.[5] Biomechanical testing of this modified technique revealed smaller prosthetic femoral head and neck angles and greater compressive medial bone strain, which is in direct contrast to the findings of a prior study.[7,26] This suggests that stress shielding may not be the primary cause for implant loosening. Implant macromotion was also noted and could potentially contribute to implant loosening in the future.[26] The investigators also suggested that a larger implant with a longer neck length could be used with the more lateral osteotomy in clinical patients to engage the lateral cortex while allowing for a greater neck angle.[26] A newer femoral neck implant design is now available in the second generation of implants, the advanced short stem (HELICA TPS stem, INNOPLANT Veterinary) (**Fig. 4**). This is a longer femoral neck implant that allows for adequate lateral cortical purchase while still maintaining a significant portion of the femoral neck.[26] The newer femoral stem design is also modular, allowing for adaptability to the individual needs of each patient.
- Another modification that has been made to the original femoral stem design is the addition of different flange sizes to increase surgical planning flexibility and improve resistance against shear forces at the interface between the implant and femoral osteotomy site.[5]

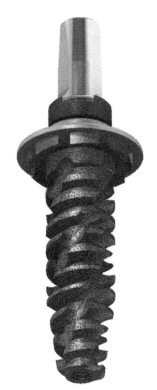

Fig. 4. HELICA TPS stem. (*Courtesy of* INNOPLANT Veterinary, Hannover, Germany.)

Clinical efficacy of these modifications has not yet been evaluated.

The screw-in femoral stem and acetabular hip endoprostheses are part of a complete THR system (INNOPLANT Total Hip Replacement system) with components that are interchangeable between the cemented and cementless systems, as the need arises (see **Fig. 2**). In addition, there are special femoral heads available (INNOPLANT Veterinary) that can be used as a hybrid on the femoral stems of the BioMedtrix or Zurich THR systems during revision surgery.

SUMMARY

The acetabular Screw Cup and HELICA TPS stem components of the INNOPLANT Total Hip Replacement are feasible options for THR in dogs. The modular screw-in cementless components can be adapted to a variety of femur sizes and may be easier to implant and require a shorter surgery time compared with other commercially available systems. Biomechanically, limitations of the first-generation screw-in implants are similar to those of other commercially available systems in small animals. Aseptic loosening is the most commonly reported complication seen after implantation whereas, to the author's knowledge, luxation has not been reported.

REFERENCES

1. Todhunter RJ, Lust G. Hip dysplasia: pathogenesis. In: Slatter D, editor. Textbook of small animal surgery. 3rd edition. Philadelphia: Elsevier; 2002. p. 2009–19.

2. Smith GK, Karbe GT, Agnello KA, et al. Pathogenesis, diagnosis, and control of canine hip dysplasia. In: Tobias KM, Johnston SA, editors. Veterinary surgery small animal. St Louis (MO): Elsevier Saunders; 2012. p. 824–48.

3. Roush JK. Surgical therapy of canine hip dysplasia. In: Tobias KM, Johnston SA, editors. Veterinary surgery small animal. St Louis (MO): Elsevier Saunders; 2012. p. 849–64.

4. Schulz KS, Dejardin LM. Surgical treatment of canine hip dysplasia. In: Slatter D, editor. Textbook of small animal surgery. 3rd edition. Philadelphia: Elsevier; 2002. p. 2029–59.

5. Hayashi K, Schulz K. Methods of immediate fixation. In: Peck JN, Marcellin-Little DJ, editors. Advances in small animal total joint replacement. Wiley-Blackwell; 2013. p. 39–51.

6. Roe SC. Implant materials: structural. In: Peck JN, Marcellin-Little DJ, editors. Advances in small animal total joint replacement. Wiley-Blackwell; 2013. p. 11–8.

7. Kim JY, Hayashi K, Garcia TC, et al. Biomechanical evaluation of screw-in femoral implant in cementless total hip system. Vet Surg 2012;41(1):94–102.

8. Hach V, Delfs G. Initial experience with a newly developed cementless hip endoprosthesis. Vet Comp Orthop Traumatol 2009;22(2):153–8.

9. Kold S, Rahbek O, Vestermark M, et al. Bone compaction enhances fixation of weightbearing titanium implants. Clin Orthop Relat Res 2005;(431):138–44.

10. Green JR, Nemzek JA, Arnoczky SP, et al. The effect of bone compaction on early fixation of porous-coated implants. J Arthroplasty 1999;14(1):91–7.

11. Windolf M, Braunstein V, Dutoit C, et al. Is a helical shaped implant a superior alternative to the dynamic hip screw for unstable femoral neck fractures? A biomechanical investigation. Clin Biomech (Bristol, Avon) 2009;24(1):59–64.

12. Peck JN, Liska WD, DeYoung DJ, et al. Clinical application of total hip replacement. In: Peck JN, Marcellin-Little DJ, editors. Advances in small animal total joint replacement. Wiley-Blackwell; 2013. p. 69–107.

13. Johnson KA. Piermattei's atlas of surgical approaches to the bones and joints of the dog and cat. 5th edition. St Louis (MO): Elsevier Saunders; 2013.

14. Olmstead ML, Hohn RB, Turner TM. A five-year study of 221 total hip replacements in the dog. J Am Vet Med Assoc 1983;183(2):191–4.

15. Bergh MS, Gilley RS, Shofer FS, et al. Complications and radiographic findings following cemented total hip replacement: a retrospective evaluation of 97 dogs. Vet Comp Orthop Traumatol 2006;19(3):172–9.

16. Liska WD. Femur fractures associated with canine total hip replacement. Vet Surg 2004;33(2):164–72.

17. Dyce J, Wisner ER, Wang Q, et al. Evaluation of risk factors for luxation after total hip replacement in dogs. Vet Surg 2000;29(6):524–32.

18. Liska WD, Poteet BA. Pulmonary embolism associated with canine total hip replacement. Vet Surg 2003;32(2):178–86.

19. Andrews CM, Liska WD, Roberts DJ. Sciatic neurapraxia as a complication in 1000 consecutive canine total hip replacements. Vet Surg 2008;37(3):254–62.

20. Guerrero TG, Montavon PM. Zurich cementless total hip replacement: retrospective evaluation of 2nd generation implants in 60 dogs. Vet Surg 2009;38(1):70–80.

21. Hummel DW, Lanz OI, Werre SR. Complications of cementless total hip replacement. A retrospective study of 163 cases. Vet Comp Orthop Traumatol 2010; 23(6):424–32.

22. Agnello KA, Cimino Brown D, Aoki K, et al. Risk factors for loosening of cementless threaded femoral implants in canine total hip arthroplasty. Vet Comp Orthop Traumatol 2015;28(1):48–53.

23. Ficklin MG, Kowaleski MP, Kunkel KA, et al. One-stage revision of an infected cementless total hip replacement. Vet Comp Orthop Traumatol 2016;29(6):541–6.
24. Andreoni AA, Guerrero TG, Hurter K, et al. Revision of an unstable HELICA endoprosthesis with a Zurich cementless total hip replacement. Vet Comp Orthop Traumatol 2010;23(3):177–81.
25. Roe SC, Marcellin-Little DJ, Lascelles BD. Revision of a loose cementless short-stem threaded femoral component using a standard cementless stem in a canine hip arthroplasty. Vet Comp Orthop Traumatol 2015;28(1):54–9.
26. Dosch M, Hayashi K, Garcia TC, et al. Biomechanical evaluation of the helica femoral implant system using traditional and modified techniques. Vet Surg 2013;42(7):867–76.

Index

Note: Page numbers of article titles are in **boldface** type.

A

Acetabular ventroversion
  JPS and, 852–854
Acetaminophen
  in CHD management, 810
Age
  as factor in CHD, 770–771
Amantadine
  in CHD management, 810
Analgesics
  in CHD management, 810
Arthroscopy
  in CHD diagnosis and evaluation, 789–790

B

Bardens test
  in CHD evaluation, 771
Barlow test
  in CHD evaluation, 771
BioMedtrix total hip replacement (THR) systems, **899–916**
  BioMedtrix Universal THR system, 902–909
  cemented *vs.* cementless implants, 900–902
  customized cementless femoral systems, 912–913
  introduction, 899–900
  Micro THR system, 909–912
  Nano THR system, 909–912
BioMedtrix Universal THR system, 902–909
Breed
  as factor in CHD, 769–770
Breeding value
  CHD screening in determination of, 802–803

C

Canine hip dysplasia (CHD)
  assessment of, **769–775**
    patient overview in, 808
    physical examination findings, 771–773
      joint subluxation tests, 771–773
      lameness evaluation, 771
      orthopedic examination, 771
  cause of, 754

Vet Clin Small Anim 47 (2017) 945–954
http://dx.doi.org/10.1016/S0195-5616(17)30049-9
0195-5616/17

Canine (*continued*)
  characteristics of, 885–886
  described, 753, 769, 807, 851, 865–866, 885, 935
  diagnosis of
    imaging in, **777–793** *See also specific modalities, e.g.,* Radiography, in CHD
      diagnosis and evaluation
    arthroscopy, 789–790
    CT, 786–787
    introduction, 777–778
    MRI, 787–789
    radiography, 778–786
    ultrasound, 786
  environmental factors and, 760–762
  etiopathogenesis of, **753–767**
  exercise and, 761
  genetics of, 758–760
  genotyping and, 759–760
  glycosaminoglycan polysulfates and, 762
  heritability of, 758
  historical background of, 823–824
  hormones and, 761–762
  introduction, 753, 795–796, 807
  joint pain with
    manual therapy, 824–825
  management of
    conservative, **807–821**
      analgesics in, 810
      chondroitin sulfate in, 812
      combination therapies in, 815–816
      complications of, 816
      corticosteroids in, 811–812
      environmental modification in, 814
      glucosamine in, 812
      hyaluronan in, 812
      introduction, 807–808
      long-term recommendations, 816–817
      neutraceuticals in, 812–813
      nonpharmacologic options in, 813–815
      NSAIDs in, 809–810
      omega-3 fatty acids in, 813
      outcome of, 816–817
      patient evaluation overview in determination of, 808
      pentosan polysulfate in, 812
      pharmacologic options in, 808–813
      physical rehabilitation in, **823–850** *See also* Physical rehabilitation, in CHD
        management
      physical therapy in, 814
      PSGAGs in, 812
      regenerative medicine in, 814–815
      rehabilitation in, 814
      weight loss pharmaceuticals in, 811

physical rehabilitation in, **823–850** *See also* Physical rehabilitation, in CHD management
surgical options in, 816
   BioMedtrix THR systems, **899–916** *See also* BioMedtrix total hip replacement (THR) systems
   femoral head and neck excision, **885–897** *See also* Femoral head and neck excision, in CHD management
   INNOPLANT THR system, **935–944** *See also* INNOPLANT total hip replacement (THR) system
   JPS, **851–863** *See also* Juvenile pubic symphysiodesis (JPS), for CHD
   physical rehabilitation after, 837–842 *See also* Physical rehabilitation, in CHD management
   TPO and DPO, **865–884** *See also* Double pelvic osteotomy (DPO); Triple pelvic osteotomy (TPO)
   Zurich Cementless THR, **917–934** *See also* Zurich Cementless total hip replacement (THR)
nutrition effects on, 760–761
pathogenesis of, 754–758
   joint laxity in, 754–755
   OA in, 756–758
   subluxation in, 755–756
prevalence of, 762–763, 795–796, 823
screening in U.S. for, **795–805**
   distraction index in, 800
   estimated breeding value, 802–803
   HEV in, 798
   improvement over generations, 802
   OFA methodology in, 796–798
   PennHIP methodology in, 798–799
   predictive value for OA development, 802
selection pressure and, 758–759
signalment of, 769–771
   age, 770–771
   breed, 769–770
   gender, 770
CHD. *See* Canine hip dysplasia (CHD)
Chondroitin sulfate
   in CHD management, 812
Codeine
   in CHD management, 810
Computed tomography (CT)
   in CHD diagnosis and evaluation, 786–787
Corticosteroids
   in CHD management, 811–812
CT. *See* Computed tomography (CT)
Customized cementless femoral systems, 912–913

D

DAR view. *See* Dorsal acetabular rim (DAR) view
Degenerative joint disease (DJD)

Degenerative (*continued*)
  JPS and, 855
Distraction index
  in CHD screening, 800
Distraction-stress radiographs
  in CHD diagnosis and evaluation, 781–785
DJD. *See* Degenerative joint disease (DJD)
Dog(s)
  hip dysplasia in *See* Canine hip dysplasia (CHD)
Dorsal acetabular rim (DAR) view
  in CHD diagnosis and evaluation, 785–786
Double pelvic osteotomy (DPO), **865–884**. *See also* Pelvic osteotomy(ies)
  bilateral procedures, 877
  clinical objectives of, 866
  complications of, 879
  degree of rotation in, 875
  implants in, 876–877
  indications for, 866–871
    hip laxity, 867–868
    joint damage, 870–871
    lameness, 866–867
    osseous conformation, 868–870
    signalment, 867
  outcomes of, 879
  postoperative period, 877–879
  rehabilitation after, 837–838
  technique, 872–874
  TPO *vs.*, 875–876
  2.5 pelvic osteotomy, 876
DPO. *See* Double pelvic osteotomy (TPO)
Dysplasia
  hip
    canine *See* Canine hip dysplasia (CHD)

  E

Environmental factors
  CHD related to, 760–762
Environmental modification
  in CHD management, 814
Exercise
  CHD related to, 761

  F

Femoral head and neck excision
  in CHD management, **885–897**
    approach to, 887
    complications of, 891
    controversies related to, 894–895

future considerations in, 894–895
  indications for, 886–887
  introduction, 885–886
  outcomes of, 893–894
  patient preparation and positioning for, 887
  postoperative care, 891–893
  technique/procedure, 887–891
Femoral head and neck osteotomy
  for CHD
    rehabilitation therapy after, 838
  sample protocol for, 846–850
Femoral overlap
  in CHD diagnosis and evaluation, 781–782

G

Gabapentin
  in CHD management, 810
Gender
  as factor in CHD, 770
Genetics
  in CHD, 758–760
Genotyping
  CHD related to, 759–760
Glucosamine
  in conservative management of CHD, 812
Glycosaminoglycan polysulfates
  CHD related to, 762

H

HEV. *See* Hip-extended view (HEV)
Hip dysplasia
  canine *See* Canine hip dysplasia (CHD)
Hip-extended radiography
  in CHD diagnosis and evaluation, 778–781
Hip-extended view (HEV)
  in CHD screening, 798
Hip laxity
  DPO and TPO for, 867–868
Hip laxity and subluxation
  JPS and, 854–855
Hip pain
  clinical measures of
    JPS and, 855–856
Hormone(s)
  CHD related to, 761–762
Hyaluronan
  in CHD management, 812

I

INNOPLANT total hip replacement (THR) system, **935–944**
    complications of, 939–940
    contraindications to, 938–939
    controversies related to, 941–942
    future considerations in, 941–942
    indications for, 938–939
    introduction, 936–937
    materials in, 937–938
    outcomes of, 940–941
    postoperative care, 940
    technique, 939

J

Joint damage
    DPO and TPO for, 870–871
JPS. See Juvenile pubic symphysiodesis (JPS)
Juvenile pubic symphysiodesis (JPS), **851–863**
    case selection for, 856
    complications of, 859
    described, 852
    effects of, 852–856
        acetabular ventroversion, 852–854
        clinical measures of hip pain and lameness, 855–856
        DJD, 855
        hip laxity and subluxation, 854–855
        OA evidence on radiographs, 855
        pelvic canal dimensions, 854
    introduction, 851–852
    radiographic characteristics of, 859–860
    rehabilitation therapy after, 837
    surgical technique, 857–859

L

Lameness
    clinical measures of
        JPS and, 855–856
    DPO and TPO for, 866–867

M

Magnetic resonance imaging (MRI)
    in CHD diagnosis and evaluation, 787–789
Manual therapy
    in CHD management, 824–825
Micro THR system, 909–912
MRI. See Magnetic resonance imaging (MRI)

N

Nano THR system, 909–912
Neutraceuticals
    in CHD management, 812–813
Nonsteroidal anti-inflammatory drugs (NSAIDs)
    in CHD management, 809–810
Norberg angle
    in CHD diagnosis and evaluation, 781–782
NSAIDs. *See* Nonsteroidal anti-inflammatory drugs (NSAIDs)
Nutrition
    CHD related to, 760–761

O

OA. *See* Osteoarthritis (OA)
OFA. *See* Orthopedic Foundation for Animals (OFA)
Omega-3 fatty acids
    in CHD management, 813
Orthopedic Foundation for Animals (OFA)
    hip/elbow database methodology of, 796–798
    PennHIP *vs.,* 799–800
        studies comparing, 801
Ortolani test
    in CHD evaluation, 772–773
Osseous conformation
    DPO and TPO for, 868–870
Osteoarthritis (OA)
    CHD related to, 756–758
        screening for, 802
    radiographic evidence of
        JPS and, 855
Osteotomy(ies)
    double pelvic *See* Double pelvic osteotomy (DPO)
    femoral head and neck
        for CHD
            rehabilitation therapy after, 838
            sample protocol for, 846–850
    pelvic *See specific types and* Pelvic osteotomy(ies)
    triple pelvic *See* Triple pelvic osteotomy (TPO)

P

Pelvic canal dimensions
    JPS and, 854
Pelvic osteotomy(ies). *See also* Double pelvic osteotomy (DPO); Triple pelvic osteotomy (TPO)
    complications of, 879
    controversies related to, 879–881
    described, 865–866
    future considerations for, 879–881

Pelvic (*continued*)
  outcomes of, 879
  rehabilitation after, 837–838
  2.5, 876
PennHIP. *See* Pennsylvania Hip Improvement Program (PennHIP)
Pennsylvania Hip Improvement Program (PennHIP)
  in CHD screening, 798–799
  OFA *vs.,* 799–800
    studies comparing, 801
Pentosan polysulfate
  in CHD management, 812
Physical modalities
  in CHD management, 835–836
Physical rehabilitation
  in CHD management, **823–850**
    after surgical management, 837–842
      femoral head and neck osteotomy, 838
      JPS, 837
      THA-THR, 838–842
      triple or double pelvic osteotomies, 837–838
    introduction, 823–824
    manual therapy to minimize joint pain, 824–825
    physical modalities, 835–836
    therapeutic exercise, 825–835
Physical therapy
  in CHD management, 814
Polysulfated glycosaminoglycans (PSGAGs)
  in CHD management, 812
PSGAGs. *See* Polysulfated glycosaminoglycans (PSGAGs)

  R

Radiography
  in CHD diagnosis and evaluation, 778–786
    DAR view in, 785–786
    distraction-stress radiographs, 781–785
    hip-extended radiography, 778–781
    Norberg angle and femoral overlap, 781–782
Regenerative medicine
  in CHD management, 814–815
Rehabilitation
  in CHD management, 814
  physical
    in CHD management, **823–850** *See also* Physical rehabilitation, in CHD management

  S

Screening
  CHD–related
    in U.S., **795–805** *See also* Canine hip dysplasia (CHD), screening in U.S. for
Signalment
  DPO and TPO for, 867

T

THA/THR. *See* Total hip arthroplasty/replacement (THA/THR)
Therapeutic exercise
  in CHD management, 825–835
Total hip arthroplasty/replacement (THA/THR)
  in CHD management
    rehabilitation therapy after, 838–842
Total hip replacement (THR)
  in CHD management *See specific types and procedures, e.g.,* BioMedtrix total hip
    replacement (THR) systems
TPO. *See* Triple pelvic osteotomy (TPO)
Tramadol
  in CHD management, 810
Triple pelvic osteotomy (TPO), **865–884**. *See also* Pelvic osteotomy(ies)
  bilateral procedures, 877
  clinical objectives of, 866
  complications of, 879
  degree of rotation in, 875
  DPO *vs.,* 875–876
  implants in, 876–877
  indications for, 866–871
    hip laxity, 867–868
    joint damage, 870–871
    lameness, 866–867
    osseous conformation, 868–870
    signalment, 867
  outcomes of, 879
  postoperative period, 877–879
  rehabilitation after, 837–838
  technique, 872–874
  2.5 pelvic osteotomy, 876
2.5 pelvic osteotomy, 876

U

Ultrasound
  in CHD diagnosis and evaluation, 786

W

Weight loss pharmaceuticals
  in CHD management, 811

Z

Zurich Cementless total hip replacement (THR), **917–934**
  approach to, 920
  complications of, 927–928
  contraindications to, 918
  controversies related to, 930–932

Zurich (*continued*)
    follow-up care, 929–930
    future considerations in, 930–932
    indications for, 918
    introduction, 917–918
    outcomes of, 930
    patient preparation and positioning for, 919–920
    postoperative care, 929
    technique/procedure, 920–927
        acetabulum preparation, 922–924
        closure, 926–927
        evaluation, 926
        femoral osteotomy, 920–921
        femur preparation, 921–922
        fixation of cup, 924–925
        fixation of stem, 925–926
        reduction, 926
        stem preparation, 924

Moving?

Make sure your subscription moves with you!

To notify us of your new address, find your **Clinics Account Number** (located on your mailing label above your name), and contact customer service at:

Email: journalscustomerservice-usa@elsevier.com

800-654-2452 (subscribers in the U.S. & Canada)
314-447-8871 (subscribers outside of the U.S. & Canada)

Fax number: 314-447-8029

Elsevier Health Sciences Division
Subscription Customer Service
3251 Riverport Lane
Maryland Heights, MO 63043

*To ensure uninterrupted delivery of your subscription, please notify us at least 4 weeks in advance of move.

Printed and bound by CPI Group (UK) Ltd, Croydon, CR0 4YY

03/10/2024

01040398-0001